Trigger Point Therapy
for Myofascial Pain

Trigger Point Therapy for Myofascial Pain

The Practice of Informed Touch

DONNA FINANDO, L.AC., L.M.T.

AND

STEVEN FINANDO, PH.D., L.AC.

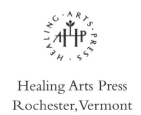

Healing Arts Press
Rochester, Vermont

Healing Arts Press
One Park Street
Rochester, Vermont 05767
www.InnerTraditions.com

Healing Arts Press is a division of Inner Traditions International

Note to the reader: This book is intended as an informational guide. The remedies, approaches, and techniques described herein are meant to supplement, and not to be a substitute for, professional medical care or treatment. They should not be used to treat a serious ailment without prior consultation with a qualified health care professional.

The Library of Congress has cataloged a previous hardcover edition of this title as follows:
Finando, Donna.
Informed touch : a clinician's guide to the evaluation and treatment of
myofascial disorders / Donna Finando, Steven Finando
p. cm.
Includes bibliographical references and index.
ISBN 0-89281-740-2
1. Myofascial pain syndromes.   I. Finando, Steven J.   II. Title.
RC927.3.F56   1999   99-25845
616.7'4—dc21   CIP

ISBN of current title *Trigger Point Therapy for Myofascial Pain*: 978-1-59477-054-8

Printed and bound in the United States by P.A. Hutchison

11

Anatomical art by Polan and Waski
Line illustrations by Jane Waski

Text design by Virginia L. Scott-Bowman
Layout by Jonathan Desautels

This book was typeset in Bembo with Italian Electric as the display typeface

◆ ◆ ◆

To our patients, from whom we have learned much about the nature

of pain and how to treat it. And to our students, who required us

to think about, order, and communicate what we practice.

CONTENTS

ACKNOWLEDGMENTS   ix

INTRODUCTION   A GATHERING OF FORCES: *Toward an Era of*
               Interdisciplinary Cooperation in the Treatment of Pain   1
CHAPTER 1   THE NATURE OF MUSCLES AND TRIGGER POINTS   3
CHAPTER 2   QI, MOVEMENT, AND HEALTH   8
CHAPTER 3   INFORMED TOUCH   19
CHAPTER 4   DIAGNOSIS AND TREATMENT   23
CHAPTER 5   HOW TO USE THIS MANUAL   29

Muscles of the Head, Neck, and Face

STERNOCLEIDOMASTOID   32
SCALENES   36
SPLENIUS CAPITIS   40
SPLENIUS CERVICIS   42
POSTERIOR CERVICALS   44
TEMPORALIS   48
MASSETER   50
PTERYGOIDS   52

Muscles of the Shoulder Girdle

TRAPEZIUS   58
LEVATOR SCAPULAE   62
RHOMBOIDS   66
SERRATUS ANTERIOR   68
PECTORALIS MINOR   72

Muscles of the Upper Limb

PECTORALIS MAJOR   78
DELTOID   82
LATISSIMUS DORSI   86
TERES MAJOR   90
SUPRASPINATUS   94

INFRASPINATUS   98
TERES MINOR   102
SUBSCAPULARIS   106
BICEPS BRACHII   110
TRICEPS BRACHII   114
BRACHIALIS   116
BRACHIORADIALIS   118
HAND AND FINGER EXTENSORS   120
HAND AND FINGER FLEXORS   124

Muscles of the Torso

ERECTOR SPINAE   130
QUADRATUS LUMBORUM   134
ILIOPSOAS   138
RECTUS ABDOMINIS   142
ABDOMINALS   146

Muscles of the Lower Limb

GLUTEUS MAXIMUS   152
GLUTEUS MEDIUS   156

GLUTEUS MINIMUS   160
TENSOR FASCIAE LATAE   164
PIRIFORMIS   168
HAMSTRINGS   172
QUADRICEPS   176
ADDUCTORS   180
PECTINEUS   184
GRACILIS   188
SARTORIUS   190
POPLITEUS   192
GASTROCNEMIUS   194
SOLEUS   198
TIBIALIS POSTERIOR   202
TIBIALIS ANTERIOR   204
PERONEAL MUSCLES   208
LONG EXTENSORS OF THE TOES   212
LONG FLEXORS OF THE TOES   216

❖ ❖ ❖

APPENDIX 1 MERIDIAN PATHWAYS   221
APPENDIX 2 ON CUTANEOUS ZONES   225
APPENDIX 3 COMMONLY USED ACUPOINTS   226

❖ ❖ ❖

PAIN PATTERN INDEX   229
SYMPTOM INDEX   237
BIBLIOGRAPHY   243

ACKNOWLEDGMENTS

*J*anet Travell, M.D., whose life work in clarifying and ordering myofascial pain syndromes has provided the reality base that has eluded so many others. Her work has demonstrated beyond any doubt that pain results from muscular dysfunction. So many in the medical community have, until very recently, disregarded the musculature as a source of pain and suffering. Through Janet Travell's lifelong work—her systematic efforts to identify and chart pain patterns associated with muscular trigger points and the various means with which to eliminate them—we have been given the basis for treatment of chronic pain suffered by so many for so long.

Mark Seem, Ph.D., who has strived to evolve the application of Dr. Travell's work to the field of acupuncture. Understanding the value of acupuncture as physical medicine in the treatment and resolution of pain, Mark has dedicated his efforts to bringing acupuncture into the forefront of American health care. We would also like to thank Mark for coining the phrase *informed touch,* which so clearly describes what we seek to accomplish through our work.

Arya Niellsen, L.Ac., Steven Rosenblatt, M.D., and Robert Ruffalo, D.C., whose feedback has helped in making this book most useful for Eastern and Western practitioners alike.

Jane Waski, whose skillful drawings demonstrate stretches that are so beautifully rendered that we can feel and sense the stretch of the muscle as we look at them.

Susan Bubenas and the staff at Polan and Waski, whose graphic capabilities have been critical in the production of illustrations that so clearly identify muscle and trigger point.

Susan Davidson of Healing Arts Press, who has helped us clarify, order, and evolve this work. Her help, her encouragement, her careful and critical editor's eye, her patience, and her dedication to this project have been invaluable to the evolution of this manual.

A GATHERING OF FORCES

*Toward an Era of Interdisciplinary
Cooperation in the Treatment of Pain*

*T*he field of pain management, specifically the treatment of myofascial pain syndromes, has become a meeting ground for health professionals. Acupuncturists, medical doctors, and practitioners of various manual and physical therapies who previously had little to say to one another are now collaborating in ways that are unprecedented in the history of American health care. The reason for the development of such interdisciplinary communication is the growing recognition that myofascial syndromes are the basis of a huge segment of patient complaint, and associated allocation of resources, within our health care system.

Patients with myofascial pain syndromes are seeking the help of family physicians, internists, orthopedists, neurologists, rheumatologists, osteopaths, physiatrists, psychiatrists, and anesthesiologists. Dentists, particularly specialists in temporomandibular joint syndrome, regularly see patients presenting with myofascial pain. In addition, acupuncturists, chiropractors, physical therapists, occupational therapists, massage therapists, and psychotherapists are all encountering patients in pain. Conferences on pain treatment have increasingly become polyprofessional experiences.

It is possible that, through health professionals' mutual interest in the treatment of myofascial pain syndromes, true complementary medicine may emerge as a reality in the United States. *Complementary medicine* here refers to the use of conventional medical practices in conjunction with recently emerging Oriental and other body-therapy approaches, providing a coordinated treatment strategy that is best for the patient. This differs from the alternative medical model, which tends toward a competitive concept of health care, ultimately forcing a division between itself and conventional medical practices that may not, in the long run, be of the greatest benefit to patients. At this point in our medical history the fact is that health professionals from widely varying disciplines are talking to each other with a new-found respect, and the result may be the fostering of a cooperative spirit that will help millions of people who are in pain.

This book, a field manual for any health professional dealing with myofascial syndromes, therefore serves a vital purpose. Its aim is to simplify and order the vast amounts of information related to the evaluation and treatment of myofascial pain. Utilizing our many years of clinical and teaching experience, we have endeavored to address the concerns and desires of health care providers for a manual that can assist in evaluating a patient, defining the presenting condition, and guiding treatment of that condition. It is assumed that the reader has some knowledge of myology; therefore no effort is made to replicate the extensive background and theoretical discussion found in seminal works on myofascial pain, such as those of Janet Travell and David S i m o n s and P. E. Baldry.* Instead, in addition to the technical core of the manual, introductory chapters discuss topics that will facilitate communication among the many professions concerned with this area of study.

We begin with a discussion on the nature of muscles and trigger points, useful as review for those who treat primarily from this perspective and a good introduction for those entering the field. We then examine the phenomenology of qi, that elusive concept of "energy" that is the foundation of all Oriental medical practices. Qi is examined from the perspective of myofascial syndromes, making it a more accessible and useful metaphor for all health professionals. It is hoped that an expanded view of the concept of qi will help facilitate, rather than hinder, communication between practitioners of Eastern and Western medicine.

Since muscle-palpation skills are at the center of effective evaluation and treatment, we next discuss the nature and process of palpation. Because a relative few practitioners are adept in this type of palpation, some guiding principles are offered to help those who are evolving palpation skills. A chapter outlining the fundamental approaches to evaluation and treatment of myofascial pain syndromes helps establish common ground among health professionals, in the realization that there are behavioral elements in treatment that are shared, independent of one's particular training or orientation. Thus the acupuncturist, neurologist, and physical therapist, while differing in perspective regarding myofascial pain syndromes, all ultimately share similar behaviors in evaluation and treatment. A brief overview of how to use the clinical body of the manual, with a description of the information provided for each muscle, finishes the introduction.

In the final analysis, since this is a manual for the health professional who encounters patients presenting with pain on a daily basis, the approach is pragmatic and behavioral. In the interest of expanding our scientific knowledge, it is enticing to determine underlying mechanisms for pain that strengthen our theoretical understanding. However, it is far more important that the practitioner in the field ascertain what helps patients, and learns how to effect that help. This book is about how, not why.

---

*Janet Travell, M.D., and David Simons, M.D., *Myofascial Pain and Dysfunction: The Trigger Point Manual,* 2 vols. (Baltimore: Williams and Wilkins, 1982–92); Peter E. Baldry, *Acupuncture Trigger Points and Musculoskeletal Pain* (Edinburgh/London: Churchill Livingstone, 1989).

CHAPTER 1

THE NATURE OF MUSCLES
AND TRIGGER POINTS

*M*ovement is a fundamental characteristic of life, and the musculature plays the major role in that activity. Motion, both gross and subtle, is an essential body function resulting from the contraction and relaxation of muscles. In humans the musculature constitutes 40 to 50 percent of total body weight. Considered as a single entity, the musculature can be regarded as the body's largest internal organ.

There are three primary functions of the muscles. First, they contribute to the support of the body and containment of the internal organs. Second, they allow movement of the body as a whole, as well as movements of the organs and substructures. Many kinds of motion rely on the integrated functioning of bones, joints, tendons, ligaments, muscles, and fascia. Both the maintenance of our upright posture as well as all body movements—walking, sitting, writing, chewing, breathing, and so forth—take place as a result of appropriate muscular activity. Internal, organic movement that is the hallmark of life relies on appropriate muscular activity: the beating of the heart and the movement of blood throughout the arterial vessels; digestion, peristalsis, and elimination; the emptying of the bladder; the very ability to draw a breath. Finally, this movement produces heat and therefore contributes to the regulation of body temperature, the third primary function of the muscles.

The three types of muscle—skeletal muscle, visceral muscle, and cardiac muscle—provide these functions. Each of these tissues exhibits four principal characteristics:

1. Excitability (irritability)—the ability to receive and respond to stimuli via nerve impulse
2. Contractility—the ability to shorten when a sufficient internal or external stimulus is received

3. Extensibility—the ability to be stretched
4. Elasticity—the ability to return to normal shape after contraction or extension

The focus of this manual is the contractile, voluntary skeletal muscle tissue. There are two types of skeletal muscle: phasic muscles and postural, or tonic, muscles.

Phasic muscles produce a contraction known as a *phasic contraction*. A phasic contraction is sufficient for the muscle to produce movement of its attachments. Phasic muscles are mainly comprised of fast-twitch fibers, which tend to produce rapid contractions and therefore function to produce rapid movements. There is a generally low capillary supply to phasic muscles and, as a result, these muscles tend to fatigue quickly. Phasic muscles tend toward the rapid accumulation of lactic acid. When there is muscular dysfunction, phasic muscles tend toward weakening.

Those that are generally considered to be phasic muscles include the midthoracic portion of the erector spinae; the rhomboids; the lower and middle trapezius; the abdominal portion of pectoralis major; triceps brachii; vastus medialis and vastus lateralis; gluteus maximus, gluteus medius, and gluteus minimus; rectus abdominis; and the external and internal obliques.

Postural, or tonic, muscles produce a sustained partial contraction of the muscle known as a *tonic contraction*. With a tonic contraction a portion of the muscle cells in the muscle are contracted at any given time while others are relaxed. This causes some contraction of the muscle; however, because enough fibers are not contracted at the same moment in time, a tonic contraction does not produce movement of the skeletal attachments.

During a tonic contraction an individual motor unit does not function continuously; rather, individual motor units within the muscle fire asynchronously, thereby relieving one another in a smooth and continuous manner. The result is a muscle contraction that can be held for long periods of time. As the name implies, these postural, or tonic, muscles act in the maintenance of upright posture; they are considered to be "antigravity" muscles. Postural muscles tend to be comprised mainly of slow-twitch fibers. There is generally a high capillary supply to these muscles, and as a result they do not tend to fatigue rapidly. Lactic acid production is minimal. When there is muscular disturbance, postural muscles tend toward shortening.

Those that are generally considered to be postural muscles include the scalenes, sternocleidomastoid, levator scapulae, pectoralis major, biceps brachii, the cervical and lumbar portions of the erector spinae, quadratus lumborum, iliopsoas, the hamstring group (biceps femoris, semitendinosus, semimembranosus), rectus femoris, tensor fasciae latae, the adductor group (adductor magnus, longus, and brevis), pectineus, gracilis, piriformis, gastrocnemius, and soleus.

Skeletal muscles, both phasic and tonic, are extremely vulnerable to injury due to overuse and the wear and tear of daily life, yet this musculature is often overlooked as a major source of physical pain and dysfunction.

In order to clearly understand the nature of an injured muscle we must first understand the qualities of normal muscle. Normal, healthy muscle tissue feels supple and elastic. The underlying structures—bones, joints, and viscera—may be easily palpated through the skeletal muscle. There is uniform consistency and plasticity within a normal muscle, and it is not tender when palpated. A healthy muscle will contract in response to nervous impulse, returning to its normal shape after contraction. Individual bundles of muscle fibers (fascicles) cannot be differentiated while palpating normal muscle.

A dysfunctional muscle will contract, but it

will not return to its normal shape following contraction. It will instead remain fixed in a shortened position, one that often results in local reduction of blood flow, lymph drainage, and range of motion. Over time a chronically contracted muscle can undergo changes in the tissue, either throughout the functional unit or within individual bands. These changes are often characterized by an increase in muscle tone, greater resistance to palpation, and decreased suppleness. Contracted musculature is no longer able to perform its activities optimally. Being shortened, it cannot perform its full range of contraction and release. Its range of motion is impaired, resulting in weakened functioning.

Taut bands, individualized bundles of muscle fiber, may be differentiated during palpation of a contracted muscle. The muscle may harbor ropelike areas, cordlike bands that can vary in thickness from thin strings to cables as much as a few centimeters thick. (Generally, bands formed in small muscles feel stringy while bands formed in larger, thicker muscles feel "ropy," or like cables.) Contracted muscle is generally reported to feel tender when mild pressure is applied. Underlying structures may be more difficult to palpate clearly, and in cases of very strong contraction, underlying structures may be completely obscured to palpation.

All of us harbor areas of constricted muscle, contracted in varying degrees, that maintain holding patterns in tight, chronically utilized muscles. These patterns can be seen in such common postural habits as holding the shoulders elevated, the chest constricted and dropped, the upper back rounded, or the lower back strongly arched. Whether due to emotional or physical patterns of overuse, our posture, our ability to move, and our ability to operate in a physiologically optimal manner are all affected by holding patterns of muscular constriction. When the constriction is chronic,

other aspects of our physiology, such as blood flow, lymphatic drainage, and nervous innervation, are eventually affected as well. Our overall health is therefore intimately related to our muscular health.

One of the many factors that may contribute to the pain and dysfunction of a muscle is the development of trigger points within it. In her encyclopedic work on trigger point therapy, Dr. Janet Travell defines a trigger point as "a hyperirritable locus within a taut band of skeletal muscle, located in the muscular tissue and/or its associated fascia."★ Myofascial trigger points—that is, those that are located in muscle (generally, skeletal muscle) or muscle fascia—are most prevalent and symptomatic; however, trigger points can also be present in cutaneous, ligamentous, periosteal, and nonmuscular fascial tissues as well. A myofascial trigger point is that area, that point, along a taut muscular band in which the tenderness reaches its maximum. The patient will feel the greatest degree of sensitivity at the trigger point; the practitioner will feel that area to have the greatest resistance to palpation (that is, it will feel like the hardest area on the taut band). A trigger point is painful upon compression. It can give rise to referred pain, tenderness, and autonomic phenomena such as visual disturbances, redness and tearing of the eyes, vestibular disturbances, space-perception disturbances, coryza (mucous membrane inflammation), reduction in local vascular activity, and skin temperature changes. The implications of such extensive effects are important in regard to the examination and treatment of many disorders that are generally not considered to be related to muscular problems.

The size of the muscle is not the characteristic that defines the degree, severity, and

---

★Travell and Simons, *Myofascial Pain and Dysfunction,* 1:12.

extent of pain caused by a trigger point within that muscle. Rather, it is the degree of hyperirritability of the trigger point that defines the degree of pain. The more hyper-irritable the trigger point, the greater the degree of pain throughout the course of the referred pain pattern.

A trigger point may begin with muscular strain or overuse that becomes the site of sensitized nerves, increased cellular metabolism, and decreased circulation. From an anatomic perspective, areas that tend to develop trigger points are generally areas in which increased mechanical strain or impaired circulation are likely to develop due to physical activities or postural stresses. Trigger points most frequently develop in the sternocleidomastoid, upper trapezius, levator scapulae, infraspinatus, thoracolumbar paraspinals, quadratus lumborum, gluteus medius, and gluteus minimus; however, trigger points can develop within any fascicle in any muscle of the body.

Trigger points can be latent or active. Both will cause stiffness and weakness of the affected muscle and restrict the muscle's full range of movement. (Stiffness is most notable after periods of inactivity, while weakness tends to be more variable.) Both active and latent trigger points are tender to palpation.

Active trigger points are differentiated from latent trigger points in that they produce pain. Therefore, active trigger points are generally considered to be of greater clinical significance. This pain tends to be referred away from the affected muscle in a character-istic pain pattern; the relationship between an active trigger point and its characteristic pain pattern has been extensively researched by Travell and Simons. There may be an abrupt onset of pain or dysfunction, whereby a specific incident is noted to be the cause of the myofascial difficulty, or the onset may be gradual, the muscle having been overloaded for some period of time. Myofascial pain may

be characterized as steady, deep, dull, and aching; it is rarely described by the patient as burning, throbbing, tingly, or numb. Pain varies in intensity from low-grade to quite severe, and it may occur at rest or in motion.

Tenderness in response to palpation can occur within the pain pattern of a trigger point even if pain is not experienced in the point's referral zone. This tenderness will dissipate after the trigger point is reduced. Pain or tenderness will generally increase with use of the muscle, stretching of the muscle, direct pressure to the trigger point, shortening of the muscle for an extended period of time, sustained repetitive contraction of the muscle, cold or damp weather, viral infections, and stress. Symptoms will decrease after short periods of light activity followed by rest, and slow, steady, passive stretching of the muscle, especially with the application of moist heat to the muscle.

Latent trigger points are far more frequent than active trigger points and are commonly found in patterns of muscular constriction that frequently define a person's "normal" posture. Latent trigger points can become active through a number of circumstances. Activation of a trigger point can occur directly through acute overload of a particular muscle, chronic overload or overwork fatigue caused by excessive or repetitive actions or sustained contraction of the muscle, trauma to the muscle, or compression or chilling of the muscle. Indirect activation can occur as a result of leaving a muscle in a shortened position for extended periods of time, as in sleeping or sitting for extended periods or holding a phone between the ear and the shoulder. Indirect activation can also result from visceral disease, viral disease, emotional stresses, or the chronic muscular strain of trying to stabilize arthritic joints, or if the latent trigger points lie within the pain pattern produced by other, active trigger points. Generally the degree of conditioning of the muscle is the factor that most defines whether a latent trigger point will become active. The greater the degree of muscle conditioning, the lower the susceptibility to trigger point activation. However, while an active trigger point will frequently revert to latency with sufficient rest, trigger points will not be fully reduced without clinical intervention.

Only adequate, focused, specific palpation techniques allow the practitioner to identify trigger points within a muscle. Through palpation we identify generalized tightness of the musculature within the vicinity of the suspected trigger point. As we palpate we locate the specific muscle that is shortened and then locate the specific band within the muscle that is taut. Continued focused palpation will reveal an area along the band that is particularly tight and then a point within the area that is exquisitely tender. Here we have located the trigger point. Direct manual pressure to that trigger point elicits what Travell called a local twitch response—that is, a literal twitch of the muscle that is sometimes visible (depending on the placement of the muscle) and is often experienced by the patient.* In addition, there may be a "patient jump sign"—that is, the patient jumps or cries out in pain.† The pain that the patient expresses is often greater than the practitioner may expect given the degree of pressure applied. With extended pressure to the trigger point, the referred pain pattern may be felt in its entirety by the patient.

Once located, the trigger point must be reduced. This is accomplished primarily through needling or through ischemic compression. Depending on the specialty of the practitioner, needling may include acupuncture needling or dry needling, or trigger point reduction techniques developed within the medical community with the use of analgesic or anesthetic injection, or the injection of saline. Ischemic compression requires compressing the trigger point for 15 to 20 seconds, followed by manipulation of the surrounding bands of muscle tissue to reduce local constrictions and taut muscular bands. Spray-and-stretch techniques, that is, the application of cold while stretching the muscle, is often helpful as follow-up to needling or ischemic compression. Treatment is completed through the application of moist heat to increase circulation to the affected muscle.

Once there is sufficient reduction of the trigger points and associated constrictions, the patient is instructed in stretching techniques specific to the involved muscles. The stretches are aimed at keeping the muscle from returning to the shortened state. Repeated stretching throughout the day is unquestionably one of the most important aspects of treatment. Finally, depending upon the degree of weakness of the muscle, after it is clear that the muscle is not readily returning to a contracted state the patient is instructed on specific strengthening exercises to help him return to optimal activity levels and to prevent the muscle from tending to return to a state of disability.

It is important to note that the conditioning of a muscle is ultimately dependent upon the conditioning of the whole body. It is vitally important to help each patient attain an optimum level of health with a program that includes exercises that will generally strengthen both the musculature and the cardiovascular system. Every part is only as viable as the whole. To view and treat a single muscle or muscle group without consideration of the whole is insufficient treatment. An expansive view of the whole body must be integrated into the care of each patient.

*Travell and Simons, *Myofascial Pain and Dysfunction*, 1:16.
†Ibid.

CHAPTER 2

QI, MOVEMENT, AND HEALTH

As acupuncturists and practitioners of Oriental manipulation therapies for over twenty-five years, our introduction to patient evaluation and treatment has been through the perspective of Oriental medicine. Unlike modern Western medical arts, Oriental medicine was developed at a time when it had neither the advantage of extensive knowledge regarding anatomy and physiology nor the burden of understanding underlying physiological mechanisms of disease and treatment. The result was a very practical medicine, refined by millennia of experience.

Years of study of Eastern philosophies have shown us how, in the ancient Orient, metaphor was used to describe the nature of the world. One of the great mistakes made by modern students of Oriental medicine and body therapies, both in the East and West, is thinking that Oriental medical principles are actual descriptors of a physical reality rather than ideas or metaphors that serve to guide treatment. In keeping with the most ancient roots of Oriental medicine, this book addresses what we, as practitioners, *do behaviorally* to effect change in the muscles and fascia, and to ultimately reduce or terminate the experience of pain for our patients. Thus, in part this manual is designed to address the following questions: How do we approach a patient who is experiencing pain? What do we look for? Where do we touch? How do we untie the myofascial Gordian knot that is so often the physical reality of one who has been in pain for an extended period of time? These are the questions that guide our approach to our patients.

Perhaps no area of Western medicine so parallels the pragmatic Eastern approach as the treatment of myofascial pain. Dr. Janet Travell, the brilliant physician who made a life's work of studying trigger points and the myofascia, was an extremely pragmatic and behaviorally oriented individual. Her careful documentation of myofascial pain patterns and associated causes and perpetuating factors represents decades of clinical experience. Without any knowledge of Oriental medicine she discovered meridian therapy in Western terms. This was a monumental feat of careful clinical observation, integrating the diverse experiences of patients in pain. Her work with Dr. David Simons, a landmark in the field, is ultimately decidedly behavioral and pragmatic in approach.[*]

On several occasions between 1991 and 1994 we had the remarkable experience of observing Dr. Travell at work; it was the opportunity to observe a master practitioner. Watching Dr. Travell treat patients was a joy. She understood what to do, where to touch, how to move, how to feel; and she ultimately helped her patients. She understood what was of benefit and hypothesized about why. The concepts and approaches that she utilized simply work; they help change lives and alleviate suffering. In our work with Dr. Travell it became clear to us that the field of pain management is one in which practices that benefit patients are shared between Eastern and Western approaches. It is curious to note, however, that practitioners of both of these systems don't really understand the nature of that which unites them.

During our first fifteen years in practice we studied and utilized both traditional Chinese medicine (TCM) and an ancient style of acupuncture that actually represents a group of methods collectively known as *meridian acupuncture*. Traditional Chinese medicine, primarily based upon an internal medical model, considers the practices of acupuncture and herbology to be inseparable. TCM emphasizes assessment through the evaluation of signs and symptoms, including the evaluation of pulse and tongue characteristics, in an effort to diagnose some internal condition.[†]

All acupuncturists study the meridians. However, unlike the practitioner of TCM, the practitioner of meridian acupuncture utilizes needles first and foremost to open constrictions along the pathways of the meridians. He generally relies on palpation skills to locate constriction, sets needles related to areas of constriction, and often identifies distal constrictions related to local ones. In practice, however, we found that the use of acupuncture techniques, both those outlined in TCM as well as those employed by meridian acupuncturists, were limited in their ability to aid patients suffering from either chronic or acute myofascial pain, regardless of the location of that pain. Neither the TCM treatments utilizing the internal medical model nor the treatments utilizing techniques based on meridian acupuncture were sufficient to completely alleviate that pain. Something was missing. When we encountered the work of Dr. Janet Travell we discovered what was clearly needed. Since that first introduction we began evolving a practice that utilizes both the Eastern perspective of meridian therapeutics and the myofascial perspective outlined so extensively by Travell and Simons. In developing this practice we perceived and treated our patients through two "lenses," and so began to see the real similarities between the patterns of pain resultant from myofascial trigger points as catalogued by Travell *and* the pathways of the meridians as they lie along the limbs and torso.[‡] By directly treating the *source* of the

---

[*]Travell and Simons, *Myofascial Pain and Dysfunction* (2 vols.).

[†]During the Cultural Revolution in China, in the midtwentieth century, acupuncture and herbal medicine were standardized, resulting in the schools of Oriental medicine all generally teaching the same curricula. That curricula was at the time named "traditional Chinese medicine." The first major translated texts on Oriental medicine came from these Chinese programs; they served as the foundation for the vast majority of acupuncture curricula taught in the United States. Within this perspective the actions of acupuncture points and the influences of herbs upon the body are generally viewed in the same way: just as certain herbs are used to reduce "intestinal heat" or alleviate "spleen dampness," certain acupuncture points are needled to assist in accomplishing the same purpose. In this approach to acupuncture, needling is practiced in order to support the effects produced by herbs; the acupuncture points are generally located by measurement or by light surface palpation.

[‡]This relationship was supported by a study performed by A. J. R. Macdonald, in which he correlated the relationship between acupuncture pathways and patterns of pain experienced by his patients suffering with myofascial constrictions. See A. J. R. Macdonald in Peter E. Baldry, *Acupuncture*, 44–45.

pain—the specific muscle harboring trigger points as identified through palpation—and then supporting that with treatment along related meridian pathways, we found that we were able to greatly alter our patients' conditions, allowing them far greater freedom from pain. Employing this integration of Eastern and Western perspectives, the work we have developed is called *myofascial meridian therapy.* This merging of Eastern and Western points of view is useful: simply put, it works.

In observing the fields of acupuncture and Oriental medicine over the past decade, we have seen unprecedented growth in the numbers of people who wish to learn about its principles and practices. These numbers include physicians, dentists, chiropractors, osteopaths, physical therapists, and massage practitioners who are seeking out additional, and perhaps more effective, means of treating their patients; as well as people who have personally benefited from acupuncture and who wish to change their career, perhaps to help others as they have been helped. In so many (if not all) cases, these people are interested in caring for the whole person, no longer satisfied with the focused specialization within the medical community in which a patient is defined by his presenting condition. Health care practitioners of all types are embracing a newfound, but old-fashioned, respect for the individual, holding a view in which a physical condition represents dysfunction within the whole and is considered within the context of its effects on the whole.

Myofascial meridian therapy is a form of treatment in which addressing a patient's pain is done within the context of treating the whole person. Because myofascial meridian therapy utilizes aspects of both Eastern and Western approaches to patient care, it can provide the basis of treatment—the meeting point—for those whose orientation lies in either Oriental medicine or allopathic medicine. Those whose background is Oriental medicine can broaden their approach to patient care and the treatment of pain by delving more deeply into the study of the myofascia, increasing their understanding of the musculature and the fascia and the complex role those play in human health and well-being. Just so, those whose background is in the Western perspectives of health care can broaden their perspective of the human experience by embracing some basic concepts utilized in the practice of Oriental medicine.

One of the most basic of those Oriental medicine concepts is that of qi, popularly conceived of as "life force." It is in the consideration of qi, redefined in Western terms, that we once again find a meeting place for both the Eastern and Western perspectives. However, in order for qi to be considered as a unifying principle for guiding treatment, its definition must be expanded and refined.

It is important to preface this discussion with the statement that Chinese philosophical concepts are extremely fluid: ideas change relative to their context and application. The point here is to provide a way in which the concept of qi may be particularly useful to the practitioner of myofascial meridian therapy, regardless of orientation. Hopefully the result will simultaneously elevate qi to a more complex concept while making its application in meridian therapies, and pain management specifically, far more pragmatic.

Perhaps the most intriguing and powerful aspect of Oriental medicine is its direct connection to universal principles. The Taoist application of cosmology to human health—the view of the human being as a part of a much broader universal system—is foundational to understanding the ancient Oriental approach to health care. Seeing the human being as a microsystem that is part of a macrosystem is intrinsic to understanding how to treat health problems. Indeed, the principles used by acupuncturists are not so much acupuncture principles as they are universal tenets applied to acupuncture.

Let us consider universal principles as described in Taoist cosmologies. Taoist cosmology begins with the idea of Wu Qi, sometimes described as Emptiness, the Void, or Nothingness. This is the universe a priori to existence. Think of what an extraordinary idea this is: it is the concept of some "thing" before anything exists. This is the idea of the unmanifest God, the Absolute, Unity, or Nirguna Brahman (in Hinduism), which refers to God without attributes. It is perhaps more accurately discussed as *a dynamic that is in perfect balance*. When there is a change in this delicate balance, some movement occurs. Movement is a relative concept—it only exists in relation to something else; therefore, movement implies duality. This is the beginning of existence, the Tai Qi, the Yin/Yang, a concept similar to the big bang theory of creation. And so we have the Wu Qi, movement as potential only, giving rise to the Tai Qi, movement made manifest in the form of duality.

Now consider the idea that, following this first movement, everything that subsequently comes into existence can only function under this universal principle of duality, Yin/Yang. All that exists is a function of, and therefore reflects, this first principle, this first movement, the beginning of duality. Existence can be viewed as a continuum of energy, starting with the highest energetic level of the Tai Qi and moving outward, slowing down, and becoming more material. The Tai Qi pervades everything, including its ultimate manifestation as the "ten thousand things," the Chinese euphemism for the material world.

Applying this idea to our work, we can therefore see that the concept of qi that is particularly useful to myofascial meridian

therapists is this notion of impetus toward movement. Organic life exists as a particular vibration, or level of movement, on this universal continuum of energy; health is intimately connected with this movement. We are not referring here to the movement of qi but rather to movement itself, with qi being the source of such movement. Qi as impetus toward movement may be equated, then, with the Tao, the "way of all things." As the Tao te Ching begins: "The Tao that can be named is not the eternal Tao."[*] If we try to name qi we have begun to bring the concept down and, in some sense, make it more "material."

Viewed from this perspective, qi is a metaphysical—rather than a physical—concept; it thus cannot be understood in physical terms or through customary language. Because language is generally developed in the context of physical reality, we are in a linguistic quandary when we enter the world of metaconcepts. Considered in this way, however, qi cannot be described or held to a specific definition, though it can be alluded to through metaphor, parable, or similar constructs. Unfortunately it is the history of such ideas to be reduced, brought down to the way we, as human beings, easily understand, and made into something physical rather than metaphysical. While the idea that qi is some sort of invisible "stuff" flowing through the meridians can have its uses, it should be understood that this is a materialized concept of qi.

The fundamental characteristic of energy is movement, and the quality and nature of this movement defines the continuum of energy and matter. This continuum can be observed by looking at water, that remarkable substance that is both the basis and the reflection of life. In its most energetic state water exists

[*]Lao Tsu, *Tao te Ching*, trans. Gia-Fu Feng and Jane English (New York: Vintage, 1972), 1.

as steam; in its least energetic and most material state it exists as ice. The metaphors of qi applied in a number of Oriental medical contexts—such as immune, muscular, and soft-tissue functions *(wei qi);* nutritive functions *(ku qi);* or genetic predispositions *(yuan qi)*—are all about harmonious movement: life connected to balanced activity; open, flowing movement. It is no wonder that qi is often connected to water metaphors (sea, river, spring, and so forth).

Conceptualizing qi in terms of movement rather than substance marries it into a philosophy of life and health held by all medical systems. Consider the words of reknowned osteopath and educator John McMillan Mennel in his discussion of the musculoskeletal system:

> The musculoskeletal system has two equally important functions. The first is movement, and the second is support (or containment). The most important part of its movement function is perhaps that *its absence is associated with death* (emphasis ours). As movement becomes more and more impaired, the functions of the systems that the musculoskeletal system is designed to contain cannot be maintained, and these other structures themselves become dysfunctional. This in itself contributes to and may hasten the final loss of function of the contained systems.*

Health requires movement; when movement ceases, life ceases. When the human organic system is functioning properly, things move well and in a coordinated, homeodynamic manner. Blood moves in a steady tidal flow, connected to such diverse and changing conditions as

muscular contraction and release, digestion, and mentation. Nerves signal through electrochemical flows in a coordinated system of activity; endocrine glands provide well-timed secretions related to the requirements of the whole. Muscles, fascia, tendons, and ligaments direct lubricated joints through complex movements. The respiratory system moves gases in coordinated quantities, while cilia and mucus provide the first line of defense against pathogens. Digestive enzymes are secreted, and harmonious peristaltic action allows for the transformation of materials into energy. Lymph is pumped and circulated as the body moves. All of this is taking place in an interactive symphony that we call life, from the cellular level to the cosmological level.

A central principle of tai qi quan holds that the universe *is* this all-pervasive movement, or activity, and it is that movement which we experience as our human bodies. Human beings are loci of this activity; the more a person is capable of relaxing, both physically and psychologically, the more he becomes a locus through which more of this movement can take place. The more constricted a person is (both physically and psychologically—which are, in fact, interdependent), the more movement is impeded. Such impediments produce consequences that affect health and well-being. Consider the words of a great taijiquan master, Dr. Jwing-Ming Yang, as he discusses the fact that many qigong practitioners mistakenly take the feeling of heat that they experience as qi:

> Actually, warmth is an indication of the existence of Qi, but it is not Qi itself. This is just like electricity in a wire. Without a meter, you cannot tell there is an electric current in a wire unless you sense some phenomenon such as heat or magnetic force. Neither heat nor magnetic force is electric current; rather they are indica-

---

*John McMillan Mennel, *The Musculoskeletal System: Differential Diagnosis from Symptoms and Physical Signs* (Gaithersburg, Md.: Aspen, 1992), 5.

tions of the existence of this current. In the same way, *you cannot feel Qi directly, but can sense the presence of Qi from the symptoms of your body's reaction to it, such as warmth or tingling* [emphasis ours].[*]

Once again we see the struggle to deal with an experience that is both physical and metaphysical. The associated warmth to which Dr. Yang refers is connected to increased circulation of blood and lymph and increased nerve conduction that occur as a result of the release that takes place during the practice of tai qi quan; that is, to the *effects* of improved movement.

Giovanni Maciocia, author of *The Foundations of Chinese Medicine,* correctly identifies the enormous difficulty in defining qi, which he describes as something that is material and immaterial at the same time. One interpretation he offers is "moving power."[†] He, like many others who have closely examined the idea, decides to leave the term *qi* untranslated.

A similar problem of definition occurs when we consider other metaconcepts, such as the idea of higher dimensions of space. Concepts such as a fourth- or fifth-dimensional space can be represented mathematically or can be discussed in metaphor (see Abbott's *Flatland* or Bragdon's *A Primer of Higher Space*[‡]), but they cannot be imaged or described. Try to picture a direction perpendicular to all three spatial dimensions (that is, image the fourth dimension), and you confront the difficulty. Qi, like other metaconcepts, is in the same category of definitional complexity. However, once we relate the concept of qi to movement, we hold a rather elegant idea that bridges Eastern and Western views of life and health.

Myofascial meridian therapy operates from this simple unifying construct. Movement, harmonious activity, unimpeded flow of bodily fluids, unimpaired nerve transmission, and the free range of motion of muscles and joints are all connected to health and life: this movement can be collectively described as qi manifesting. Constriction, impingement, entrapment, ischemia, and excessive tightness, all associated with dysfunction and pain, can thus be considered in terms of some reduction in movement. Be it of an organ, muscle, fluid, or electrochemical impulse, with pathology there is some interference with flow, with movement, with qi. Death is the result of its ultimate withdrawal.

Given the functional definition of qi as movement, myofascial meridian therapy is concerned not with "moving" some substance called qi, *but rather with removing or minimizing disruptions to movement itself.* Our inclination is to trust the inherent wisdom of the body; we endeavor to provide an optimum environment in which the body can heal itself. Therefore it is the role of the myofascial meridian therapist to release constrictions and promote flow. While the fundamental approach is myofascial, the broad concepts and patterns of the meridian system are also embraced. The successful release of myofascial constriction comes from applying knowledge and understanding of these meridian patterns in conjunction with the ability to palpate and release constrictions within the muscular and fascial systems.

Diagnosis, therefore, is intimately associated with treatment, since the diagnosis is neither of internal diseases or patterns of disharmony as theorized from an Eastern perspective nor the expression of Western medical pathologies.

---

[*]Jwing-Ming Yang, *Tai Chi Theory and Martial Power* (Jamaica Plain: YMAA, 1987), 27.

[†]Giovanni Maciocia, *The Foundations of Chinese Medicine* (Edinburgh/London: Churchill Livingstone, 1989), 36.

[‡]Edwin A. Abbott, *Flatland: A Romance of Many Dimensions* (New York: HarperCollins, 1983); Claude Bradgon, *A Primer of Higher Space* (London: Kessinger, 1999). Originally published 1939.

Rather, to diagnose from a myofascial meridian perspective the practitioner palpates the body to locate patterns of constriction and then uses acupuncture or manual techniques to release these constrictions. Principles of Oriental medicine guide the direction of care.

Myofascial meridian therapy is concerned with constriction not only in the muscles but also in the fascia. The fascia is unique in human physiology, existing as a single continuous sheath that extends from the head to the toes, encasing every organ, muscle, and muscle fiber as it winds through the body. Consider the definition of fascia as proposed by Dr. William Henry Hollinshead:

> When the normal connective tissues of the body are arranged in the form of enveloping sheaths, they are usually known as **fasciae** (fascia means a bandage or band, and thus connotes a layer binding together other structures). Thus, the subcutaneous tissue or tela subcutanea is frequently called the *superficial fascia*. Numerous examples of well developed, tough, deep fasciae occur, especially in the limbs, where fascia forms heavy membranes surrounding the entire limb. Individual muscles are also surrounded by thin fascia called perimysium and are separated from each other by looser connective tissue. . . . From the fascia surrounding a muscle, connective tissue septa pass into the muscle and subdivide it into bundles; these septa, in turn, divide until delicate connective tissue fibers surround each muscle fiber within a muscle.★

The superficial fascia covers the entire body subcutaneously. It is composed of two layers: the outer layer contains fat; the inner layer is thin and elastic. Lying between the layers of superficial fascia are the arteries, veins, lymphatics, mammary glands, and facial muscles. The deep fascia lines the body wall and the extremities; it holds the muscles together and separates them into functional groups. Deep fascia allows for the movement of muscles. It assists in support and stabilization, aiding in the maintenance of balance. It carries nerves and blood vessels, fills spaces between the muscles, and sometimes provides attachments for muscles. Fascia facilitates circulation of the lymphatic and venous systems. Differentiation of the deep fascia begins with the envelopment of the individual muscle by the epimysium, the external sheath of connective tissue. The epimysium further differentiates into the perimysium, the fascia that wraps bundles of muscle fibers (fascicles), and this further differentiates into the endomysium, which penetrates the interior of each fascicle to enwrap each muscle cell. This system is continuous with the structure of tendons that attach muscle to other structures.

Doctor of osteopathy John Upledger describes the fascia as "a maze which allows travel from any one place in the body to any other place without ever leaving the fascia."† Fascia's pervasive, continuous nature may explain many of the distal effects of acupuncture or other meridian-based forms of bodywork. Paula Scariati, D.O., observes that changes in the fascia due to age or trauma "set off chain reactions that may compromise the vasculature, nervous system and muscle as well as change the movement of body fluids through the fascia."‡ It logically follows, then, that if constriction of fascia can produce dys-

---

★David B. Jenkins, *Hollinshead's Functional Anatomy of the Limbs and Back,* 6th ed. (Philadelphia: Saunders, 1991), 12.

†John Upledger and Jon Vredevoogd, *Craniosacral Therapy* (Seattle: Eastland, 1983), 239.

‡See Paula D. Scariati, "Myofascial Release Concepts," in *An Osteopathic Approach to Diagnosis and Treatment,* eds. Eileen L. DiGiovanna, D.O., and Stanley Schiowitz, D.O. (Philadelphia: Lippincott, 1991), 365.

function, the release of constriction within the fascia can lead to a return of function.

There has been much speculation on the functional mechanism of acupuncture; much has been made about the activation of beta-endorphins, a powerful pain supressant, resulting from acupuncture treatment. Actually, the experience of any systematic minor pain will give rise to the inhibitory response of endorphins—pinching the skin anywhere will produce endorphins. It is conceivable that endorphin activity is a pleasant secondary effect of acupuncture treatment and is unrelated to the mechanism that underlies its more powerful effects.

It is more probable that the answers to the question of how acupuncture works lie in the study of the little understood and complex mechanisms that govern the fascia, muscles, skin, and adipose tissue of the body. The fact that dramatic releases of muscular constriction can be affected by surface needling is well documented by Travell and Simons on a muscle-by-muscle basis. Such release is also capable of exerting powerful visceral effects. The probability of understanding acupuncture lies in the reality of what is actually being done to the patient: a needle is being inserted into tissue, and such insertions and manipulations have extensive local and distal effects.

Ultimately we should consider the simple fact that, in the realm of acupuncture treatment and bodywork, practitioners insert needles or apply manual-therapy techniques to skin, adipose tissue, fascia, and muscle. Significant effects are exerted by such treatment. Practitioners can say they are manipulating qi by treating points on the meridians, but they cannot deny that they are also manipulating skin, adipose tissue, fascia, and muscle.

What is the difference? Why make an issue about qi? Consider this perspective: Rather than moving some invisible, untouchable "substance" (that is, qi), *treatment of the skin, muscle, fascia, and adipose tissue opens constrictions and promotes the movement of all bodily functions and activities.* The point is to focus our attention, and therefore to focus our skills, on what we definitely can and do affect: physical structures, such as the muscles and fascia. Just as qi cannot be experienced directly, in a model where qi cannot be manipulated directly the increase in movement, or flow, occurs as a consequence of releasing myofascial constrictions. The easing of myofascial restriction therefore results in improved circulation, lymphatic drainage, and nerve conduction. Additional results may include improved organ function (such as lung tidal volume, digestive activity, or uterine function), depending upon the location of release. Such focus on myofascial constriction, instead of on qi, allows for a shift of perception to a readily identified source of pain or pathology, which, when released, results in improvement of the condition.

These basic tenets of such a physical medicine underlie treatment effects that go beyond pain management. This is best understood by considering the somatovisceral and viscerosomatic reflex connections—that is, the relationships between the soma (the musculature) and the viscera (the organs), a phenomenon recognized by the fields of osteopathy and chiropractic and utilized in their diagnoses and treatments. The *somatovisceral reflex connection* is defined as muscular disruptions that alter the ability of related visceral organs to function properly. These are situations in which myofascial constriction directly results in visceral symptoms such as tachycardia, angina pectoris, diarrhea, vomiting, food intolerance, and dysmenorrhea. (The phenomenon of somatovisceral effects is also discussed in detail by Travell and Simons.) Conversely, the *viscerosomatic reflex connection* is defined as dysfunction of the myofascia resulting from disease or dysfunction of a related visceral organ. When applying the basic principle of myofascial meridian therapy, the identification and release of patterns of myofascial constriction includes but is not limited to the release of trigger points in individual muscles. Myofascial meridian therapy involves the release of a region, a quadrant, and ultimately the complete body. This leads to freedom of movement throughout the organism on multiple levels, superficially as well as deeply, directly or indirectly affecting the viscera and resulting in improved health.

Clearly this physical approach to diagnosis and treatment differs from the traditional Chinese medical model in that the prominent use of herbs parallels the use of pharmaceuticals in Western conventional medicine; neither has proven to be markedly effective in treating chronic and acute myofascial pain. This failure lies in the inability of such medications, Eastern or Western, to focus on the central issue of these patterns of pain. Acupuncture and associated bodywork therapies, when utilized as myofascial meridian therapies, *do* in fact focus on the central issues of movement and constriction, and as a result have demonstrated that their greatest power lies in their specifically physical approach.

Many within the conventional medical establishment have noted the often remarkable effects of acupuncture and bodywork therapies on patients who suffer from chronic pain. Herein lies the source of increased communication among practitioners. Medical doctors are beginning to recognize the difficulties in the medical/surgical approach to treatment of chronic pain and are viewing, with greater respect, meridian acupuncture and bodywork therapies as effective *physical* treatment methodologies.

Meridian therapies are based upon the palpatory experience. The exacting nature of myofascial meridian therapy requires enormous emphasis on palpation, with the therapist evolving great skill in identifying myofascial constrictions. The charts of meridians and acupuncture points are used as general maps of areas where specific loci may be identified. Locating acupuncture points is thereby not a function of measurement but rather of palpation, connected to the skill of the practitioner's hands. The points are moving realities that shift on the body landscape. Everything about our bodies is dynamic, moving, changing; in the same way, acupuncture points exist as dynamic rather than static entities. The focus is therefore on constriction, on the real and present reality— treatment decisions are based not on cerebral or intellectual construction but on the practitioner's palpatory experience. Because a fundamental component in the evolution of palpation skill is the ability to visualize and understand what you are feeling with your hands, a working knowledge of the meridian system is necessary and a careful study of anatomical structure, with an emphasis on myology, becomes crucial.

In the practice of myofascial meridian therapy, assessment and treatment happen differently than they do within the Western medical model. Treatment within the conventional medical model focuses on the administration of a drug to effect a change in the symptoms experienced by the patient, without regard for myofascial constrictions that may accompany the symptoms. For example, it is not uncommon for a patient who is suffering with a digestive disorder, such as esophageal reflux, irritable bowel syndrome, or chronic constipation, to be prescribed a medication without attention being given to concurrent myofascial constrictions. This is not to suggest that medications are unnecessary; however, it is becoming increasingly clear that medications are often overutilized to the exclusion of other treatment methodologies from which the patient may also benefit. Using the myofascial meridian therapy model, diagnosis follows not only from the description of the pathology as experienced by the patient, but also from the practitioner identifying associated myofascial constrictions. Treatment is focused on releasing those myofascial constrictions through needling or through manual techniques.

Successful treatment of a patient who presents with irritable bowel syndrome will thus involve the therapist releasing areas of muscle and fascia that commonly relate to such bowel symptoms, and may in fact be reflections of the bowel symptoms—these areas include the rectus abdominis and external obliques. Utilizing principles rooted in the ancient Oriental texts, treatment might also include needling or massaging areas of the Hand Tai Yang Small Intestine and Hand Yang Ming Colon meridians, which pass along the posterior aspect of the shoulder and thus coincide with the infraspinatus and posterior deltoid. Palpation of this region may identify constrictions within local musculature, which would then be treated with needling or manual techniques. This approach to irritable bowel syndrome might therefore also result in improved movement of the shoulder and arm.

Additionally, in assessing the patient the therapist might note a "tautness" or "fullness" associated with the tissues overlying the tibialis anterior muscle distal to the knee, which coincides with the pathway of the Foot Yang Ming Stomach region that is associated with its Hand Yang Ming Colon pair. Treatment by needling or manual techniques to these areas will result in reduction of fullness or a softening of the tautness. The result of this treatment will likely be a deeper, more complete release of tissues leading to an improvement in the patient's overall condition. The therapist is guided by such relationships.

Myofascial meridian therapy embraces the concept of qi in a manner that focuses on a clear and present palpable reality: *If Qi is lifeforce and lifeforce is movement, then Qi is movement.* This model of qi and how it relates to health has a number of distinct advantages over an herbalized acupuncture or bodywork that first and foremost regards pathology from an internal medical model. First, this model of qi is clearly understandable to both patients and other health care practitioners. The focus of treatment is on myofascial release by extremely effective means; and while the mechanism may not be fully comprehended, the concepts of somatovisceral effects and referred pain patterns can be readily understood, particularly once the pathways of the pain patterns are pointed out on pain pattern charts. The effects of this approach are also easily explained, since the rapid myofascial release produced by a needle contacting the fascia or trigger points is well documented by Travell and others, as are the effects of ischemic pressure. Through experience in treatment the effects are also clearly observable, to patient and practitioner alike.

It is also important to recognize that this model falls well within a complementary medical model rather than an alternative medical approach. By and large myofascial meridian therapy is complementary to Western medicine, which does not focus on myofascial problems and associated release of constrictions; often the medical approaches to myofascial constriction, which include medications or surgical intervention, produce unsatisfactory results. Herbal medicine, like Western medicine, is another form of internal medicine. It is alternative to the conventional Western medical model, rather than complementary.

Certainly regarding qi as movement is not

the only way to conceive of qi within the framework of Oriental medicine. The fluidity and relativity of the philosophical constructs that underlie Oriental medicine require that ideas such as this one be examined in relation to their applications. Acupuncture and associated bodywork methods have enormous power to heal in a manner that is distinct and separate from internal medicine applications—

this is observed repeatedly in a clinical setting. This power can be actualized within an approach that looks at qi in a way that is useful and practical.

Models are ideas that help to frame reality in a complex world, and thereby allow some effective action to be taken. They are not *the* Truth, but *a* truth that guides activity.

CHAPTER 3

INFORMED TOUCH

*I*t is currently estimated that at some point in their lives approximately 90 percent of all Americans will experience some sort of myofascial pain—back pain, shoulder pain, neck pain, elbow pain—that has its roots in some dysfunction of the musculoskeletal system.

Regardless of method, the successful treatment of myofascial pain disorders ultimately rests on a singular skill. This is the ability to palpate, the ability to discern our patients' needs through touch.

Since the rise of modern technological health care, surface palpation has been the skill most overlooked in the training of health professionals. Palpation of the musculature—assessment through touch of the muscles, tendons, and fascia—is a fine and discerning art, one that is becoming lost in the morass of technologies now applied to health care. The health professions have generally forgotten the effectiveness of touch in both determining the extent of patients' pains and disabilities and in the treatment and resolution of that pain. Through palpation we can discriminate normal, supple musculature from musculature that is constricted or contains trigger points; palpation can also assist in discerning the source of myofascial pain. Our hands tell us about the alignment of the joints, about skin and body temperature, and about the flow of life on the body's surface. When trained well, our hands can "see" the structures that underlie the skin: the muscles, skeletal structure, and organs. In myofascial work the hands are our greatest tool, as long as we train them to the nuances of touch perception and learn to use them properly.

Training of the hands begins with bringing awareness to them. Practice placing your awareness in your hands. The ongoing effort to intentionally connect your mind to your hands is the key to successful training. This is not only true when touching the body, but when touching anything, all day long. Touch with attention—all touch explorations begin with this new focus. For specific exercises in palpation see Leon Chaitow's *Palpatory Literacy* (see bibliography).

The second essential requirement for the development of excellent palpation skills is the presence of a clear mental image of the structures being palpated. This requirement cannot be emphasized enough. You must be able to clearly visualize the anatomic structures of the human form as you try to palpate them; it is therefore necessary to study the anatomy of the musculoskeletal system. A keen knowledge of skeletal structure and the attachments, fiber direction, and function of each muscle is essential. Begin with knowledge, the idea, and the image, and then train your hands to "see" what you know is there.

It is important to recognize that the qualities of musculature exist on a continuum. Hypotonic or flaccid muscle, that is, muscle that has reduced tone, lies on one end of this continuum; hypertonic or excessively constricted muscle lies on the other. What you feel within any given muscle will fall anywhere within this continuum. Healthy muscle tissue is soft, supple, and resilient to pressure. The underlying structures are easily palpated through such muscle. Muscle tissue that is healthy is pain-free when palpated.

As you move through the continuum you will encounter muscle that is somewhat tight, not as resilient to the touch as supple muscle. This tissue feels harder and tougher than surrounding musculature, and a stronger, firmer touch is required to palpate the underlying structures. Firm palpation may produce some discomfort in the patient. This type of muscle we call *constricted muscle*.

The degree of constriction is dependent upon the muscle's state of contraction. When a muscle is held in a partially contracted position, groups of fibers that form the muscle may be identified and discerned. There may be taut bands of tissue within such muscle. These taut bands may feel thready or ropelike—not unlike a small cable; they can feel resistant to pressure and be somewhat uncom-

fortable to the patient when pressed. In addition, through palpation you might identify a particular region within the taut band that the patient experiences as particularly sore to the touch. To the practitioner this region feels more constricted, harder, than the areas immediately adjacent to it along the band. This region characterizes what Travell and Simons have termed a *trigger point*. When a trigger point is palpated it can cause significant local discomfort in the patient. In addition, pressure to the point can initiate the characteristic radiating pain pattern charted by Travell and Simons and others. This radiating pain is the distinguishing characteristic of trigger point activity within the myofascia.

In contrast to the partially contracted muscle just described, a deeply contracted muscle is one that remains in the muscle's extreme contracted position. This contracture may be the result of neurological dysfunction, chronic structural imbalances, trauma, or extreme repetitive strain. In cases of contracture, circulation to the muscle is reduced, and as a result the muscle becomes more fibrous, losing its elasticity. The muscle becomes fixed in a shortened position. Trigger points may or may not be present; pain and dysfunction will more likely be due to loss of full range of movement. The condition will be chronic and complete recovery improbable. With practice the practitioner can discern these various characteristics of the musculature.

When palpating it is essential to identify and differentiate skeletal structures under your hand. This ability is an essential prerequisite to muscular palpation. Locating and differentiating the bony structure will provide the structural awareness to image, first with your mind and then with your hands, the attachments of muscles to be palpated.

The ability to clearly identify a muscle under one's hand (for example, differentiating the deep thoracic paraspinal muscles from the more superficial trapezius and rhomboids) is often contingent upon the practitioner's ability to follow the course of the muscular fibers. Herein lies another reason for knowing bony landmarks by touch—it is difficult to feel for fibers and fiber directions when there is no awareness of where the muscles attach. An awareness of fiber direction in both superficial and underlying musculature is necessary to evolve the skill of differentiating muscular layers. In addition, it is important to have a working knowledge of other structures that might be within the region being palpated, such as lymph nodes in the anterior and posterior triangles of the neck and in the femoral triangle.

Attentive practice will provide you with the skill that is desired—and that is truly required—to understand the dysfunctions causing pain and discomfort to your patients. Skilled hands not only can ascertain the muscle or muscles that are involved, but as you follow constricted muscle fibers through their course you can arrive at an image of the habitual physical postures your patient assumes that could be the source of the myofascial problem. For example, in palpating his neck and shoulders you may "see" with your hands that the left side is considerably more relaxed than the right: the right sternocleidomastoid is contracted, the right trapezius is contracted, and the right levator scapulae is contracted. What posture could this person be taking to produce this muscular configuration? He might possibly be sitting in front of a computer with the monitor off to the left instead of directly in front of him. Perhaps he elevates his right shoulder in directing his cursor around the computer screen. Maybe his television at home sits to the left of his favorite chair. At least you have a mental image, an initial clue, a place from which to question your patient to find out what his habitual activities might be. Knowing the muscular action, knowing the postural habits and feeling the muscular configurations, allows you to do effective detective work. You are then able to help your patient change his habits in order to alleviate perpetuating factors giving rise to his difficulties. This discernment is essential to helping the patient rectify the muscular problem.

To palpate most effectively, the following basic principles should be embraced and practiced:

1. Clearly image the area to be palpated.
2. Soften and relax your fingers, hands, and arms in order to make full, firm contact with the area under palpation.
3. As you palpate, use as broad a surface area of your hand as possible. Palpation, as a method of gathering information, is far more effective if practiced using the palmar surfaces of the hands rather than the tips of the fingers. In using a broad hand you cover more "ground" and can thus evolve a clearer mental image of the area under palpation.
4. Identify pertinent bony structures in the region.
5. Palpate each muscle in at least two directions:
    - along the muscle fiber, from its proximal to its distal attachment, to locate the muscle and identify its size and shape; and
    - across the muscle fibers, to isolate areas of constriction, taut bands, and trigger points.
6. Limit pressure to the point of muscle resistance. When you feel the muscle providing some resistance to pressure, keep your contact at that level of pressure. Deep, excessive pressure that causes some pain will produce an automatic tightening of the body and will prevent you from clearly identifying underlying

structures; pressure that is too light will not allow you to contact the muscle properly, and a great deal of information will be overlooked as a result.

7. Palpate each muscle bilaterally to provide direct comparison. Remember that bilateral musculature should optimally be equally soft and supple and have the same shape and form. By comparing sides you can easily note areas of constriction that may exist in one side and not the other.

In summary, palpation is an essential diagnostic and treatment tool that requires attentive practice, an ability to clearly visualize musculoskeletal anatomy, and a state of relaxation that helps maximize information-gathering skills. It is through extensive clinical practice that one can evolve a clear sense of the continuum of myofascial states and an understanding of the habits of action that are the source of an enormous percentage of pain syndromes.

It is important to remember that when a patient experiencing pain is touched by a practitioner in the "right" places, a level of trust develops immediately, alleviating a great deal of the patient's fears and tension. This alone provides enormous therapeutic benefit. It begins with understanding hands, with informed touch.

CHAPTER 4

DIAGNOSIS AND TREATMENT

*I*t is assumed that the reader of this book has some experience in working with myofascial pain. However, a few basic ideas, perhaps known in some disciplines but not in others, may serve as common ground in delineating a broad protocol for the diagnosis and treatment of myofascial disorders.

Spend some time looking at the patient. Observe how he or she walks, stands, sits, breathes, holds his hands, crosses his legs, reads intake forms, rubs his neck, carries a purse, backpack, or briefcase. These and myriad other behaviors provide clues regarding the nature of his condition. While some patients will have difficulty identifying the sites or patterns of their pain, the observant clinician can learn a great deal by paying close attention to this person who has come for help. It is rare that muscular constrictions and trigger points exist in an isolated, single muscle. Careful attention can reveal a great deal about the unique and often complex pattern presented by each patient. Watching how the patient rises from a chair, gets on or off a treatment table, removes a coat, or wears out his shoes can provide valuable information leading to the effective treatment of his complaint. As in many medical therapies the clinician must be part detective, developing an ability to pick up on these clues, since they can be as important as any diagnostic testing procedure.

We had the privilege of watching Dr. Janet Travell treat a number of patients. She began formulating her treatment the moment she saw the patient enter the room. She took note of the person's shape, size, asymmetries, gait, posture, and the many ways he was holding himself, particularly when in pain. When the patient pointed out his problem, Dr. Travell was already aware of the muscular patterns involved—the history expanded the data she had already collected through observation. Before Dr. Travell touched the patient she knew a great deal about him; in fact, after fifty years of clinical experience she was so integrated in her awareness that she often saw the problem in seconds.

Dr. Travell trained herself as a better clinician with each patient she treated, which left us with another tenet for good practice: Do not assume that you know anything. Be it through palpation or questioning, in every treatment with every patient *always* seek more information about the problem (and the person) at hand.

Evolve palpation skills. Through touch the patient discovers much about the nature of the practitioner. That first touch tells the patient whether you are gentle or rough, respectful or invasive, careful or careless, and most importantly, if you know what you are doing. It is a good idea to first palpate the area where the patient is complaining of pain, since it demonstrates, in a matter of seconds, that you understand that he or she has pain and that the pain is there, where you are palpating. So often patients will exclaim, "That's it," and with those two words they have begun to accept and trust you as a practitioner. As the practitioner explores related areas the patient will often remember pains or injuries that were not mentioned in his medical history. It is as if the palpation examination opens new doors in the patient's understanding of his own problem and encourages him to come to some insight regarding the direction of treatment.

Palpation is an art and a skill. It requires work, practice, and the constant awareness that you are touching a *person*, not just a muscle. As most myofascial problems involve sequences of numerous associated muscles, effective examination will generally involve extensive palpation around the area of most acute presentation. In acupuncture, a common assessment principle has the practitioner examine left and right, up and down, and front and back relative to the presenting region. This simply means that if a patient is complaining of pain in the left lumbar region,

examination should include the right lumbar region, the upper back and shoulders, the buttocks and legs, and the abdomen. Such wide examination not only renders significant information but also respects the patient as a whole person.

Learning to touch another person includes awareness that the body will often tense to "guard" itself against invasive touch, particularly in painful areas. Such responses mitigate effective palpation, so the practitioner must learn *how* to touch, gradually applying pressure and earning the trust of his patients to allow for accurate palpation.

Regardless of the particular method of treatment employed, skillful palpation is the defining factor differentiating highly successful practitioners from those who obtain erratic results. Regardless of theory, method, or amount of treatment, skillful palpation is without question the singular most important component of treatment.

Listen closely. First, the patient has direct experience of the problem. His descriptions of what he feels and when and how he feels it are extremely important pieces of data. Second, many patients with chronic pain have suffered the experience of being told that the pain is "in their head" or "isn't real." They will often feel they have to convince you of the reality of their experience. Listening and confirming their reality is important in developing the trust necessary for treatment. Educating patients about the nature of myofascial pain syndromes, showing them wall charts of pain patterns, describing postures and movements that can trigger pain patterns as well as what kinds of organic dysfunctions might be associated with such syndromes is important. We have seen patients lose their tension and anxiety as soon as they saw their pattern on a wall chart; many have exclaimed, "I'm not crazy!" This kind of confirmation and education goes a long way in establishing a relationship that leads to effective treatment.

Additionally, it is important to remember and respect the subjective nature of the experience of pain. What might seem to be a mildly constricted area to your touch can in fact be a source of considerable pain to the patient. As you listen to your patient, hear him and embrace his reality.

Treat with precision and attention. The following approach to patient care is designed to help to focus in on the problem at hand and its resolution.

1. Clearly define the areas of pain and restrictions of movement that the patient is experiencing. Have him delineate, and perhaps draw, the areas of the body that feel painful. Have him demonstrate the movements that cause pain. Be certain that you understand, to the best of your ability, what he is experiencing.

2. Determine the various muscles that might be the source of your patient's pain and restriction. Utilizing the pain pattern and symptom indices (see pages 229–242) will be useful in this determination.

3. Palpate for constrictions and taut bands in the individual muscles that you have hypothesized to be the source of the difficulty.

4. Palpate associated regions for additional constrictions and taut bands. It is important to palpate the entire body, anterior and posterior, to determine associated constrictions. Additionally, awareness of the pathways of meridians and cutaneous zones will provide a guide for identifying restrictions that might lie outside of the affected quadrant.

5. Locate individual taut bands in the involved muscles. "Capture" the band with precise palpation and compression.

Define the specific trigger point along the taut band through focused palpation.

6. Apply treatment to the trigger points. Once the bands and trigger points are captured, maintain pressure through ischemic compression until softening of the point occurs. This can be used for treatment in and of itself; however, if acupuncture needling is used, lightly peck the point until you feel a softening of the band under the hand that is compressing the muscle. Palpation of the region after treatment will provide feedback as to whether or not there has been a complete release of the muscle.

Repeat this process of treatment with each area of constriction in each region that you identified as having restrictions. This is an essential component in obtaining complete release.

7. Apply moist heat. Whether in the office or at home, moist heat should be applied to the treated regions to increase blood flow to the areas. This should be done for at least twenty minutes each day for three days following treatment.

8. Provide a stretching program. Once the patient has had moderate release of muscular constrictions, instruct him in appropriate stretching exercises to maintain the release of the muscle. These should be done several times a day. Performance of the stretch should not produce pain.

9. Provide a strengthening program. When the patient has been pain free for seven to ten days, instruct him in appropriate strengthening activities, if the muscle needs reconditioning.

10. Teach your patient how to breathe.

Poor breathing patterns connected to stress, muscular problems, or respiratory trauma can directly affect myofascial problems. The single biggest offender is paradoxical breathing, a phenomenon in which the movements opposite to those required for a full, relaxed breath occur. Instead of the abdominal muscles relaxing in order for the contracted diaphragm to fully enlarge the thoracic cavity, the abdominals contract and the chest lifts, inhibiting the tidal volume of the lungs. Watch a patient breathe and you may notice a raising of the chest and pulling in of the abdomen. Many people reflexively do this when they try to hold the breath. It is simply incorrect breathing and often nothing more than a bad habit.

Since it can be a perpetuating factor for a number of pain syndromes, as well as part and parcel of many stress-related disorders, this type of breathing should be corrected.*

The following exercise can help retrain breathing patterns.

1. Direct the patient to sit or stand with the body naturally erect and yet relaxed. Keep the spine elongated and allow the musculature and the surrounding bony structure—the shoulders and rib cage—to relax and drop down toward the pelvic region. Allow the chest to relax; let the muscles of the abdomen and stomach relax. Let the buttocks and lower abdomen relax.

2. Take a slow breath, allowing the musculature of the stomach and abdomen to expand somewhat with the breath. Breathe in this way for a few moments, allowing the breath to move down into the lower portions of the thorax. As constrictions of abdominal and/or thoracic musculature are felt, intentionally relax the area. If the chest or shoulders rise up, return to the focus of dropping the breath into the lower areas of the body.

3. Now inhale deeply. Allow the musculature of the thorax to relax. As the musculature relaxes the chest will expand slightly in an anterior direction, in a lateral direction, and in a posterior direction. This will happen naturally in the relaxed body. Sense that a container is being filled: first the lower portion fills, then the upper portion.

4. Now exhale, emptying the upper portion first and then the lower portion. Allow the body to deflate as a balloon deflates; it will do so evenly—anteriorly, posteriorly, and laterally.

5. Relax the breath and continue to breathe fully and completely, paying attention to the pitfalls: the shoulders may want to rise up, the abdominal muscles may tighten. Keep them relaxed.

6. Instruct the patient to practice in front of a mirror at first. The reflection might demonstrate what is not yet felt—the chest rising, not dropping; the abdomen pulling in, not relaxing out.

7. Practice. Learning requires successful repetition over time.

Extend treatment beyond the office. Your job goes beyond releasing myofascial constrictions and trigger points. The treatment of myofascial pain is multifaceted and includes involving the patient in home care, such as applying moist heat; attending to postural, visual, work habit, or sleeping corrections; addressing stress management and nutritional considerations; correcting sports movements; or even suggesting new arrangements for furniture and computer stations. We often have asked patients to bring their bicycles or tennis racquets to the office if we suspected such activities were directly connected to the generation of their pain. The

---

*Travell and Simons identify potential effects related to syndromes of the abdominals, pectoralis minor, scalenes, serratus anterior and posterior, and sternocleidomastoid muscles.

clinician as detective, one who sorts out and identifies the perpetuating factors associated with the patient's condition, is only one of the roles we must assume. We must also be educators, prodding parents, or sometimes simply friends who care about the fact that a person is in pain. Familiarity with simple exercises, nutritional considerations, stress management techniques, breathing exercises, methods of changing eye-dominance, and furniture and exercise-equipment ergonomics is part of the diverse knowledge necessary for treating myofascial pain in a complete sense.

Soften the dichotomy between treatment and examination. From the outset the practitioner should view examination as treatment and treatment as examination. Failing to recognize the ongoing feedback involved in this process can result in the loss of important information. As you gather information by palpating the myofascial constriction, you are engaged in treatment. Just so, as you seek to release myofascial constrictions, you are engaged in evaluation. The act of treatment can show you the correctness of your palpation, the reactivity of the muscle, the extent of the problem, and possibly the approximate length of time this muscle has experienced distress. Further, each release can guide you to associated areas of constriction. Watching the skin surface and carefully feeling for the type and direction of the release provides evaluative information that directs the course of treatment. The patient will often describe loci of pain that are experienced at the time of palpation or treatment that correlate with the referred pain pattern, though he might also describe a distal location, demonstrating additional muscular constriction. Evaluation, treatment, and treatment planning are processes that occur simultaneously in working with myofascial pain syndromes. Therefore a certain mental framework—a diffuse state of

attention coupled with a constant vigilance that records cues and transforms them into treatment modifications—is central to this approach. Such activity becomes part of a practiced process that is carried out in treatment.

While a diagnosis is made after the history is taken, the examination is finished, tests are reviewed, and palpation is completed, it should be considered preliminary. The treatment of myofascial pain problems is also diagnosis. Whether you are injecting trigger points, releasing tender points with acupuncture, applying ischemic pressure, or performing a spray-and-stretch technique, all procedures reveal further information about the patient's condition. Attention to how the muscles respond, how the pain is experienced, the nature of the fasciculations, and how the patient responds to treatment are all pointing to the next steps of treatment. To make a firm diagnosis and carry out a rigid treatment plan is contradictory to the experience of interacting with myofascial problems. This is a world where as muscle fibers release others may constrict; where simple movements could drastically affect a recently released, but highly reactive, muscle. It is a world that is so interconnected it is impossible to understand one muscle in isolation from the whole body. The successful practitioner understands this deeply and engages in a practice that involves a kind of passive vigilance and fluidity of thought that allows for constant change. The idea that X, and X alone, is the problem and that Y will fix it is a classic error common in health care but disastrous in the world of treating myofascial pain.

John Upledger has referred to the fascia as "a single and continuous laminated sheet of connective tissue . . . [which] extends without interruption from the top of the head to the tips of the toes. It contains pockets which allow for the presence of the viscera, the visceral cavities, the muscles and skeletal structures."* The complex, interactive nature and homeodynamic activity of this system must be appreciated and respected.

As practitioners we have come to experience a fundamental state of awe that is with us each day as we treat our patients. The complexity and beauty of the myofascial system has led us to experience some amusement when a patient, learning of the nature of his or her condition, remarks, "You mean it's *just* muscular?" Exactly. It's *just* the Grand Canyon.

---

*Upledger and Vredevoogd, *Craniosacral Therapy*, 237–38.

CHAPTER 5

HOW TO USE THIS MANUAL

*T*his manual provides important information in a format that can be easily and quickly accessed by both the student and the working health care practitioner, making it readily useable in the clinic or office.

In the technical body of the book an illustration of each muscle and the locations of its common trigger points is accompanied by the following information:

Proximal attachment: The cephalad (upper) attachment, that is, the attachment closest to the head.

Distal attachment: The caudad (lower) attachment, that is, the attachment farthest away from the head.★

Action: What the muscle moves, the purpose of its action.

Palpation: Specific instructions on how to locate and palpate the muscle, including anatomical landmarks for reference.

Pain pattern: An illustration of that muscle's essential pain pattern is accompanied by a written description that also details possible extended pain patterns. Symptoms produced by the presence of trigger points in the muscle are also described.

Causative or perpetuating factors: A description of common behaviors that either produce or perpetuate the pain.

Satellite trigger points: Additional muscles and muscle groups that commonly develop trigger points when there are trigger points in the muscle.

Affected organ systems: Due to the relationship between skeletal muscle and meridian pathway, the constriction of each muscle or muscle group will

---

★Following in the work of Dr. Janet Travell, attachments of the musculature have been described in terms of proximal attachment and distal attachment rather than origin and insertion. We have opted for this description due to the effect of many muscles on both locations of attachment, making the terms *origin* and *insertion* inaccurate descriptors.

affect the meridian pathway traversing it. As each meridian exercises influence over a specific organ or system, this section may shed additional light on the interaction between skeletal muscle and viscera.

Associated zones, meridians, and points: A statement of other areas predisposed to muscular constriction when there are trigger points in a particular muscle, to guide treatment for those practicing from an Oriental medical perspective. For a review of meridian pathways and zone description, see appendices 1 and 2.

Stretch exercises: Illustrations and descriptions of stretching exercises useful for that particular muscle. Varying levels of stretch exercises may be provided to patients to accommodate their changing capacities during the healing process.

Strengthening exercises: A description of useful strengthening exercises for the muscle and associated muscle groups. A strengthening exercise is included for phasic muscles, which tend toward weakening. Tonic, or postural muscles, tend toward shortening, making strengthening exercises generally unnecessary.

Regarding the trigger point illustrations, it must be remembered that they serve only as a means to guide the initial palpation, since trigger points can present at any point in any muscle.

Most patients present with symptoms that are usually described as a particular pattern of pain. Some patients will also present with other symptoms, such as impaired range of motion, usually described as an inability to perform particular tasks. Other symptoms might seem less related, such as dizziness or menstrual problems. Two indexes are provided in an effort to help the practitioner quickly focus his or her attention on muscle groups that commonly relate to the pain pattern or symptoms presented by the patient.

The Pain Pattern Index is a graphic index in which the pain patterns for each muscle are illustrated. The pain patterns are grouped in terms of the area affected: pain patterns that affect the neck are shown together, pain patterns that affect the anterior legs are shown together, and so on. With this information ready comparisons of patterns can be made and specific information about the muscle groups quickly located.

Some patients may be vague about their pain but clear on other symptoms. The Symptom Index provides common symptoms of myofascial syndromes and the page numbers of related muscles.

Using the indexes to help narrow the focus to particular muscles involved, then turning to the summary information for each muscle, should help guide examination, treatment, and follow-up with the patient.

This manual is designed for quick access for use in clinical situations. The material is meant to supplement and guide the careful taking of case history, examination, and palpation, not to replace them.

This manual does not outline each muscle of the body. The muscles that have been included are those that we have found to be the most clinically significant in our years of practice. Pain experienced by the great majority of patients may be alleviated through the treatment of these muscle groups. For an indepth discussion of each muscle in the body, use of *Myofascial Pain and Dysfunction: The Trigger Point Manual* (volumes I and II) by Travell and Simons is recommended.

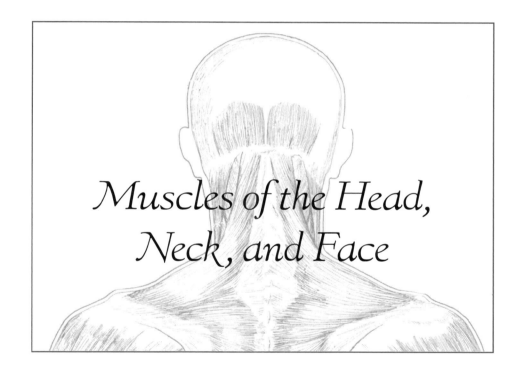

Muscles of the Head, Neck, and Face

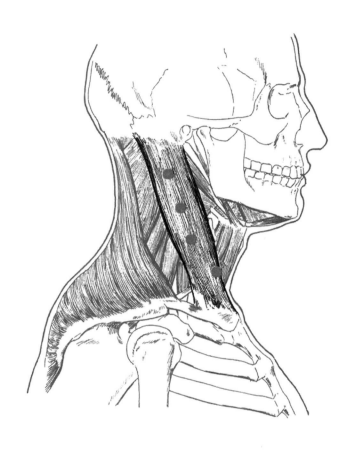

Sternocleidomastoid and trigger points

STERNOCLEIDOMASTOID

Proximal attachment: Mastoid process and the lateral half of the superior nuchal line of the occipital bone.

Distal attachment: *Clavicular head:* superior border of the anterior surface of the medial one-third of the clavicle. *Sternal head:* anterior surface of the manubrium, medial and more superficial than the clavicular head.

Action: *Acting unilaterally:* rotation of the face to the opposite side and lifting the chin; aids in sidebending to the same side. *Acting bilaterally:* flexion of the head and neck; checkreins backward motion of the head during chewing; auxillary muscle of inspiration.

Palpation: To locate the sternocleidomastoid (SCM), identify the following structures:

- Mastoid process—Follow the base of the occiput toward its lateral edge. The rounded, most lateral prominence is the mastoid process.
- Clavicle—Follow the curved course of the clavicle, from its articulation with the sternum to its articulation with the acromion. Medially the contours of the clavicle are convex; laterally its contours are concave.
- Sternoclavicular articulation—Locate the suprasternal notch at the superior aspect of the manubrium. Move laterally to locate the sternoclavicular articulation. Note that the clavicle is raised slightly above the manubrium at the articulation. By raising and lowering the shoulder as you palpate the articulation, you can clearly distinguish between the manubrium and the clavicle.
- Transverse process of C1—Locate the angle of the mandible, the sharp, lateral aspect of the jawbone. Moving posteriorly, the bony prominence of the transverse process of C1, lying between the angle of the mandible and the mastoid process, may be palpated on some people. Palpate bilaterally, gently, as this area may be quite tender.

To palpate the sternocleidomastoid, begin at the mastoid process with the patient lying supine. Locate the thickened proximal aspect of the SCM. Use your index finger to border the muscle's medial aspect and your ring finger to border its lateral aspect. Place your middle finger along the belly of the muscle and follow it down to the attachments on both the manubrium and the clavicle. Tilt the chin up toward the opposite side to differentiate clearly between the sternal attachment—thin and cordlike at its insertion—and the broader, flatter clavicular attachment on the upper surface of the clavicle.

It is interesting to note that the SCM and the trapezius have a continuous attachment along the base of the occiput. This attachment splits at the mastoid process. They have a noncontinuous attachment along the superior border of the clavicle.

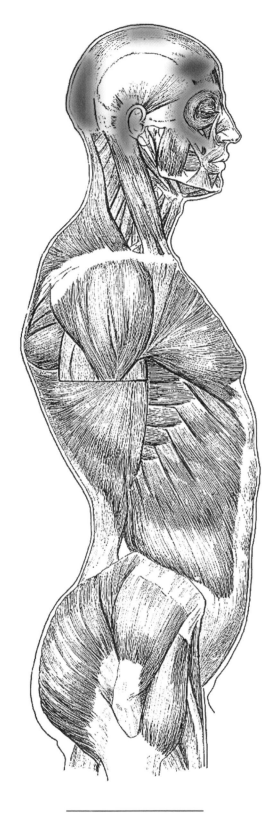

Sternocleidomastoid pain pattern

Pain pattern: *Clavicular head:* Pain refers to the frontal area—when severe, it extends across the forehead to the opposite side. Homolateral pain deep in the ear. Symptoms are frontal headache, dizziness, and postural imbalance. *Sternal head:* Cheek, temple, and orbit pain; pain that arches across the cheek and into the maxilla, over the supraorbital ridge. Vertex pain with scalp tenderness. Symptoms include dry cough and autonomic phenomena of the eye, including tearing and redness.

Causative or perpetuating factors: Mechanical overload in extension or flexion; chronic rotation to one side; whiplash; compression of the neck; paradoxical breathing or chronic cough.

Satellite trigger points: Contralateral SCM, scalenes, levator scapulae, trapezius, splenius cervicis, sternalis, pectoralis major.

Affected organ systems: Respiratory system; eyes, ears, throat; nasal sinuses.

Associated zones, meridians, and points: Ventral and lateral zones; Foot Yang Ming Stomach meridian; ST 10, 11, and 12; CO 17 and 18; SJ 16; SI 16.

Stretch exercises:
1. *Clavicular head:* Bend head and neck backward, rotating the face to one side. The muscle will be stretched at the clavicular head on the opposite side.
2. *Sternal head:* Turn head to one side, then at full rotation tilt the chin toward the shoulder. The muscle will be stretched at the sternal head on the same side.

Strengthening exercises: Isometric against mild forward resistance.

1. Place the palm heel on the forehead for resistance. Press the forehead into the resistance.
2. Clasp the hands behind the head, just below the crown. Press the head and neck posteriorly, against the resistance.

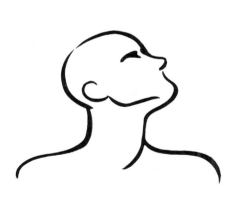

Stretch exercise 1: Clavicular head

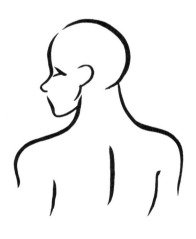

Stretch exercise 2: Sternal head

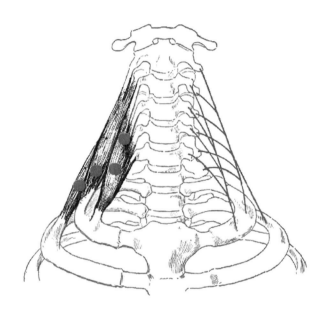

Scalenes and trigger points

SCALENES

Proximal attachment: Transverse processes of C2–C7.

Distal attachment: *Anterior and medius:* first rib. *Posterior:* second rib.

Action: *Acting unilaterally:* lateral flexion of the cervical spine. *Acting bilaterally:* stabilization of the cervical spine against lateral movement; elevation of the first and second ribs to assist in inspiration.

Palpation: To locate the scalenes, identify the following structures:

- Thyroid cartilage—Located along the anterior midline of the neck. The superior border of the thyroid cartilage, the Adam's apple, lies anterior to C4; the distal border of the thyroid cartilage lies anterior to C5. The thyroid cartilage can be observed moving up and down during swallowing.
- Hyoid bone—Located above the thyroid cartilage and lying horizontally. The hyoid bone is the first bony structure to be palpated as you move downward along the midline from the mandible. It can be palpated as it moves up and down during swallowing. The hyoid bone lies anterior to C3.
- External jugular vein—Begins near the angle of the mandible, crossing the sterno-cleidomastoid in the superficial fascia before passing posterior to the posterior border of the muscle, to empty into the subclavian vein. In the healthy patient, lying supine, the vein is clearly visible only a short distance above the clavicle. However, with increased thoracic pressure (noted in pathologies such as heart failure, enlarged supraclavicular lymph nodes, and obstruction of the superior vena cava) the external jugular vein becomes prominent throughout its course.
- Sternocleidomastoid muscle—See muscle description on page 33.

The scalenes can be palpated when they are constricted or harbor trigger points. Note the location of the external jugular vein where it crosses the sternocleidomastoid: constriction of the anterior scalene can be palpated just deep to this area. Move the palpating finger slightly posteriorly to this area to locate the scalenes; they will feel like taut bands if they are constricted.

It is essential to palpate this area with the greatest sensitivity to patient tenderness and discomfort. An extremely gentle touch is required to be able to palpate the muscle without causing pain to the patient.

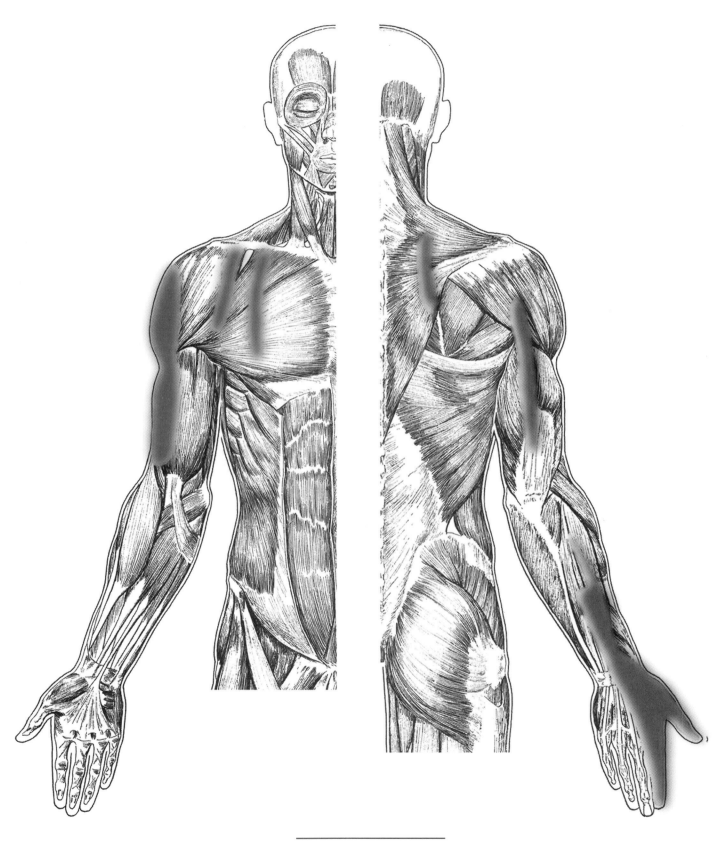

Scalenes pain pattern

Pain pattern: Persistent, aching pain that radiates anteriorly and downward toward the chest in fingerlike projections and/or laterally to the upper arm. Pain may skip the elbow and reappear at the radial side of the forearm, hand, thumb, and index finger. Pain may radiate posteriorly into the midscapular area.

Causative or perpetuating factors: Paradoxical breathing; chronic cough; pulling or lifting, especially with the arms level with the waist; chronic rotation of the cervical spine to one side.

Satellite trigger points: Sternocleidomastoid, upper trapezius, levator scapula, splenius capitis, pectoralis major, triceps.

Affected organ system: Respiratory system.

Associated zones, meridians, and points: Ventral zone; Foot Yang Ming Stomach meridian; SI 16.

Stretch exercise: Laterally bend the head and neck so that the ear of the unaffected side moves toward the same shoulder. Hold for a count of ten. Then, without changing the degree of lateral stretch, rotate the head and face toward the affected side, stretching the cheek toward the ceiling. Hold for a count of ten.

Return the head and face to the initial lateral stretch position. Now rotate the head and face, this time aiming the chin in toward the clavicle. Hold for a count of ten. Return the head and face to the initial lateral stretch position.

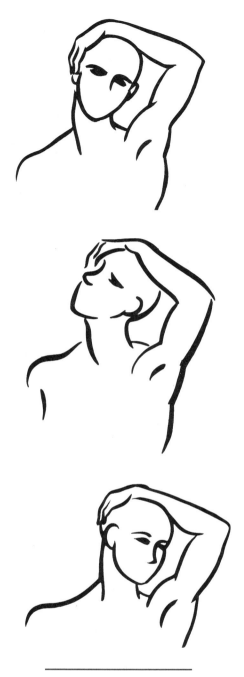

Stretch exercise: Scalenes

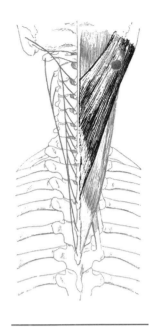

Splenius capitis and trigger point

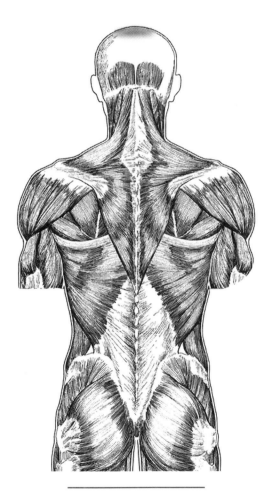

Splenius capitis pain pattern

SPLENIUS CAPITIS

Proximal attachment: Mastoid process and adjacent occipital bone, deep to the attachment of the sternocleidomastoid muscle.

Distal attachment: Fascia in the midline over the spinous processes of C4–T4.

Action: *Acting unilaterally:* rotation of the head and neck to the same side. *Acting bilaterally:* extension of the head and neck.

Palpation: To locate splenius capitis, identify the following structures:

- Sternocleidomastoid—See muscle description on page 33.
- Trapezius—See muscle description on page 59.
- Levator scapulae—See muscle description on page 63.

To palpate splenius capitis, place your patient in the seated position with his back resting on the back of the chair, or lying supine. Palpate the portion of splenius capitis that lies just above the angle of the neck: locate the muscular triangle that is formed by the sternocleidomastoid muscle (anteriorly), the trapezius muscle (posteriorly), and the levator scapulae (distally). Gently palpate taut bands of splenius capitis just proximal to the levator scapulae.

Pain pattern: Pain located at the vertex of the head.

Causative or perpetuating factors: Postural stresses that overload, such as thrusting the head forward to compensate for excessive thoracic kyphosis.

Satellite trigger points: Levator scapulae, upper trapezius, sternocleidomastoid, splenius cervicis.

Affected organ system: Vision.

Associated zones, meridians, and points: Dorsal zone; Foot Tai Yang Bladder meridian.

Stretch exercise: Rotate the head 20 to 30 degrees toward the unaffected side. Gently press the head forward and toward the unaffected side, stretching slightly more forward than laterally.

Strengthening exercise: Isometric against mild posterior resistance. Clasp the hands behind the head at the level of the nuchal line. Press the head and neck posteriorly against the mild resistance provided by the clasped hands.

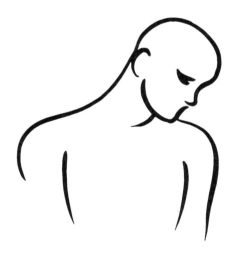

Stretch exercise: Splenius capitis

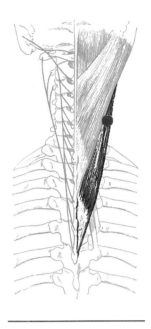

Splenius cervicis and trigger point

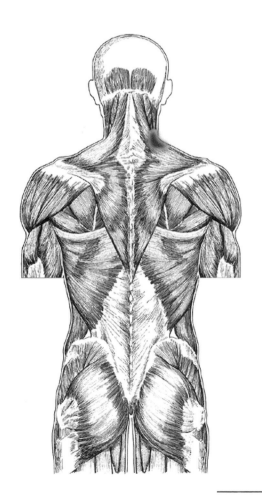
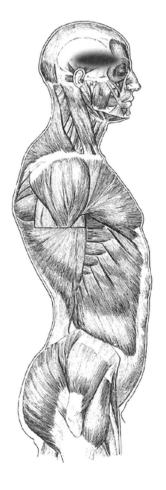

Splenius cervicis pain pattern

SPLENIUS CERVICIS

Proximal attachment: Posterior tubercles of the transverse processes of C1–C3.

Distal attachment: Spinous processes of T3–T6.

Action: *Acting unilaterally:* rotation and side-bending of the neck. *Acting bilaterally:* extension of the neck.

Palpation: To locate splenius cervicis, identify the following structures:

- Trapezius—See muscle description on page 59.
- Levator scapulae—See muscle description on page 63.

To palpate splenius cervicis, place your patient in the seated position with his back resting comfortably on the back of the chair. Laterally bend the patient's head slightly to the side being palpated, thereby relaxing both the trapezius and the levator scapulae. Palpate with one or two fingers on the vertical plane that exists between the trapezius and the levator scapulae, moving the trapezius posteromedially and the levator scapulae anterolaterally. Gently rotate the patient's head slightly to the opposite side. Palpate taut bands vertically within the defined space.

Pain pattern: Pain in the neck, cranium, and eye; patient may experience stiff neck associated with the pain. Upper trigger point causes aching pain through the head to the back of the eye on the same side, with a possible blurring of vision in that eye. Lower trigger point causes pain radiating upward and to the base of the neck.

Causative or perpetuating factors: Postural stresses that overload, such as thrusting the head forward to compensate for excessive thoracic kyphosis.

Satellite trigger points: Levator scapulae, upper trapezius, sternocleidomastoid, splenius capitis.

Affected organ system: Vision.

Associated zones, meridians, and points: Dorsal zone; Foot Tai Yang Bladder meridian.

Stretch exercise: Drop the head forward, rotating the neck 30 to 40 degrees to the side. Gently press the head down, more forward than lateral. The muscle on the opposite side will be stretched.

Strengthening exercise: Isometric against mild posterior resistance. Clasp the hands behind the head at the level of the nuchal line. Direct the patient to press the head and neck posteriorly against the mild resistance provided by the clasped hands.

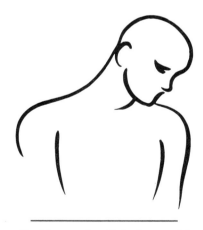

Stretch exercise: Splenius cervicis

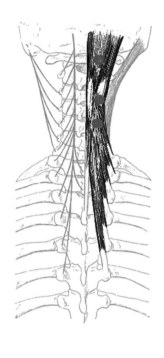

Posterior cervicals and trigger points

POSTERIOR CERVICALS

SEMISPINALIS CAPITIS AND SEMISPINALIS CERVICIS

Proximal attachment: *Semispinalis capitis:* on the occiput between the superior and inferior nuchal lines. *Semispinalis cervicis:* spinous processes of C2–C5.

Distal attachment: *Semispinalis capitis:* transverse processes of T1–T6; articular processes of C3–C7. *Semispinalis cervicis:* transverse processes of T1–T6.

Action: *Acting unilaterally:* slight rotation of the neck to the contralateral side (semispinalis cervicis) and slight rotation of the head and neck to the same side (semispinalis capitis). *Acting bilaterally:* extension of the neck (semispinalis cervicis) and extension of the head and neck (semispinalis capitis).

Palpation: Semispinalis capitis is considered to be one of the most powerful muscles of the neck. Palpate the posterior cervicals simultaneously. Semispinalis cervicis lies deep to semispinalis capitis.

To locate the the posterior cervicals, identify the following structures:

- Occiput—The base of the skull
- Spinous processes of C2–C5

Palpate semispinalis capitis through the superficial musculature of the neck. With the patient lying supine, locate the base of the occiput, supporting it with the palms of your hands. Palpate with the pads of the second, third, and fourth fingers, moving distally from the occiput toward the lower cervical region. Place your hands with your fingers lying in the direction of the long fibers of the muscles, adjacent to the spinous processes of the cervical vertebrae. Your fingers will be covering the region under which semispinalis capitis lies beneath the more superficial trapezius and splenius muscles. Deep, flat palpation will note thickened areas of muscle approximately 2 centimeters ($^3/_4$ inch) wide. Constrictions may be noted approximately 1 to 2 inches below the occiput and at the level of C4–5.

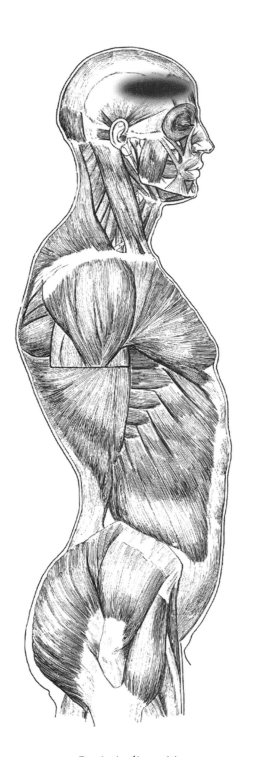

Semispinalis capitis

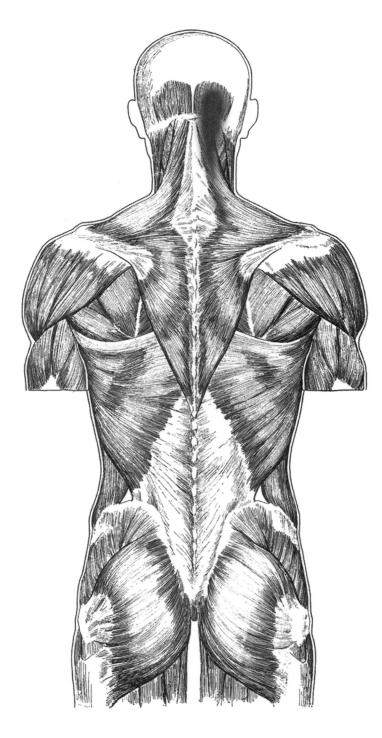

Semispinalis cervicis

Posterior cervicals pain pattern

Pain pattern: Proximal trigger point refers pain that encircles the head, reaching its maximum intensity at the temple and forehead over the eye. Intermediate trigger point refers pain over the occiput and toward the vertex. Distal trigger point (C4–5 area) refers pain and tenderness to the suboccipital region and down over the neck and upper part of the shoulder girdle. Symptoms include pain in the neck; restriction of head and neck flexion, with possibly some restriction of head and neck rotation and extension; and tenderness at the back of the head and neck.

Causative or perpetuating factors: Sustained flexion of the neck (semispinalis cervicis) and of the neck and head (semispinalis capitis); sustained extension of the neck and head.

Satellite trigger points: Bilateral posterior cervical muscles.

Affected organ system: Vision.

Associated zones, meridians, and points: Dorsal zone; Foot Tai Yang Bladder meridian; BL 10–17.

Stretch exercise: Drop the head forward, aiming the chin for the chest. Allow the weight of the head, acting with gravity, to stretch the posterior neck muscles. In doing so the chin will reach the lowest possible level on the chest. It is important to try to avoid pulling the chin in toward the throat during this stretch.

Strengthening exercise: Isometric against mild posterior resistance. Clasp the hands behind the head at the level of the nuchal line. Press the head and neck posteriorly against the mild resistance provided by the clasped hands.

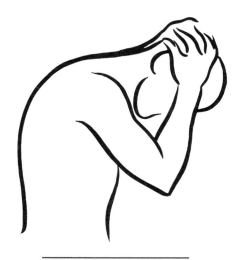

Stretch exercise: Posterior cervicals

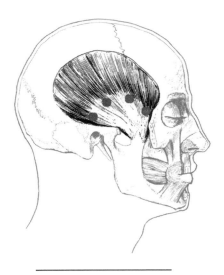

Temporalis and trigger points

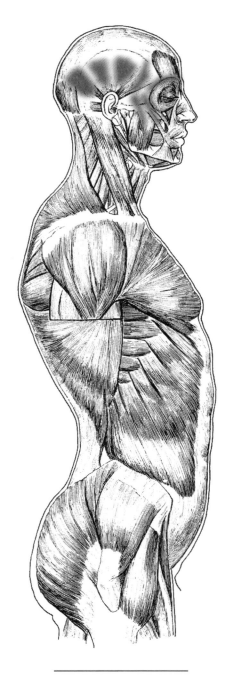

Temporalis pain pattern

TEMPORALIS

Proximal attachment: Lateral skull in front of and above the ear in the temporal fossa.

Distal attachment: Coronoid process of the mandible.

Action: Elevation of the mandible, closing the jaw; posterior fibers act in retraction of the mandible. *Acting unilaterally:* deviation of the mandible to the same side.

Palpation: To locate the temporalis, spread the fingers across the muscle just posterior to the temples and above the ears. Gentle compression of the rear teeth will produce contraction of the muscle, which will be easily experienced under the palpating hand

Palpate temporalis moving caudal to its attachment at the coronoid process of the mandible. With the mouth relaxed and open, identify trigger points in various portions of the belly of the muscle using a cross-fiber palpating technique. Trigger points that occur at the junction of the muscle fibers and its distal attachment may be found approximately 1 inch above the zygomatic arch.

Pain pattern: Temporal headache and maxillary toothache. Pain extends over the temporal region to the eyebrow, the upper teeth, and occasionally to the maxilla and the temporomandibular joint (TMJ). Trigger points can refer pain, tenderness, and hypersensitivity of the upper teeth to hot, cold, and pressure. Patients rarely complain of restricted jaw movement.

Causative or perpetuating factors: Excessive forward head posture; overuse of the muscle due to gum chewing, jaw clenching, or bruxism; chronic overuse due to an anteriorly displaced temporomandibular joint disc; direct trauma to the muscle caused from a fall or impact to the side of the head; secondary to trigger points in the sternocleidomastoid or upper trapezius.

Satellite trigger points: Contralateral temporalis, ipsilateral masseter, trapezius, sternocleidomastoid.

Affected organ system: Digestive system.

Associated zones, meridians, and points: Lateral zone; Foot Shao Yang Gall Bladder meridian; GB 3–7.

Stretch exercise: Spread the fingers across the muscle, just posterior to the temples and above the ears. Open the mouth as wide as possible and inhale. On the exhale, press upward along the fibers of the muscle.

Strengthening exercise: Due to the nature of this muscle, strengthening exercises are not necessary.

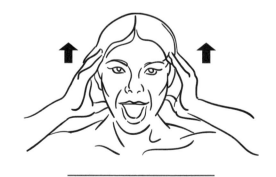

Stretch exercise: Temporalis

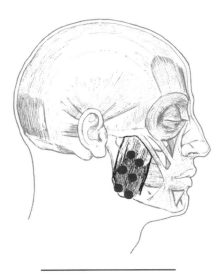

Masseter and trigger points

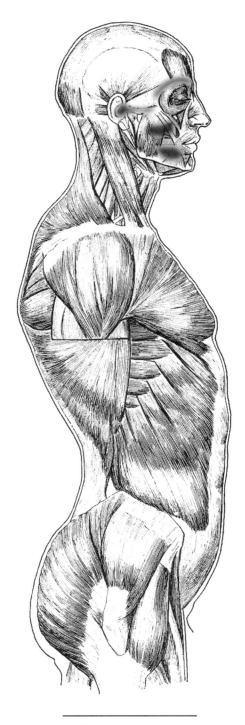

Masseter pain pattern

MASSETER

Proximal attachment: *Superficial layer:* anterior two-thirds of the zygomatic arch. *Deep layer:* posterior one-third of the zygomatic arch.

Distal attachment: *Superficial layer:* external surface of the mandible at its angle and the inferior half of the ramus of the mandible. *Deep layer:* lateral surface of the coronoid process of the mandible and the superior half of the ramus.

Action: Elevation of the mandible, closing the jaws.

Palpation: Palpate masseter with teeth slightly separated and the jaw relaxed. Beginning just below the zygomatic arch, palpate muscle fibers distally toward the angle of the mandible. Gently compressing the teeth will aid in the identification of masseter; however, the presence of the parotid gland may hinder clear identification of muscle fibers. Palpate on the inside of the cheek with a gloved hand. Place one finger within the mouth and another on the outside of the cheek to support the palpating thumb. Using cross-fiber palpation, locate taut bands of masseter.

Pain pattern: *Superficial layer:* Pain at the upper teeth and cheek, sometimes identified as sinus pain; pain at the lower teeth and jaw, above the eyebrow, and at the region of the temporomandibular joint (TMJ). *Deep layer:* Pain in the cheek and TMJ area deep in the ear; patient may experience unilateral tinnitus that is not associated with loss of hearing or vertigo and/or a marked restriction of mouth opening. Unilateral trigger points produce restricted mouth opening with deviation to the ipsilateral side. Symptoms include sensitivity to pressure, heat, and cold; restricted jaw opening. (Normal jaw opening will allow the comfortable insertion of the knuckles of two stacked fingers into the mouth.)

Causative or perpetuating factors: Forward head posture; chronic mouth breathing; acute overload from forcible contraction of the masseter as might occur while biting something quite hard; bruxism, clenching, gum chewing, nail biting; occlusion difficulties that might be resultant from the loss of natural teeth or ill-fitting dentures; psychological stresses; over-stretching that might occur with dental work; trauma from a blow to the head; chronic infection; as a satellite trigger point to sterno-cleidomastoid or upper trapezius.

Satellite trigger points: Temporalis, medial pterygoid, contralateral masseter.

Affected organ system: Digestive system.

Associated zones, meridians, and points: Lateral zone; Foot Yang Ming Stomach meridian; ST 5 and 6.

Stretch exercise: Ask the patient to slowly open the mouth against mild resistance placed on the lower jaw. Hold against light resistance for a count of three to five. Repeat three times. Following this stretch cycle, open and close the mouth several times without resistance. Note: This may be used as a trigger point release technique as well as a stretch exercise for the patient.

Strengthening exercise: Due to the nature of this muscle, strengthening exercises are not necessary.

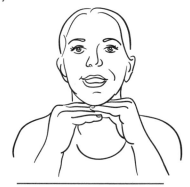

Stretch exercise: Masseter

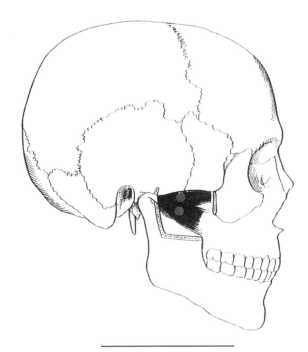

Lateral pterygoid and trigger points

PTERYGOIDS

MEDIAL (INTERNAL) PTERYGOID AND LATERAL (EXTERNAL) PTERYGOID

Proximal attachment: *Medial pterygoid:* medial surface of the lateral pterygoid plate of the sphenoid bone; the maxillary tubercle. *Lateral pterygoid:* lateral surface of the lateral pterygoid plate of the sphenoid bone; the greater wing of the sphenoid at the base of the skull.

Distal attachment: *Medial pterygoid:* medial (inner) surface of the ramus and angle of the mandible. *Lateral pterygoid:* the neck of the mandible below the condyle and the joint capsule and articular disc of the temporomandibular joint.

Action: *Medial pterygoid:* elevation of the jaw. *Acting unilaterally:* lateral deviation of the mandible to the opposite side (producing grinding motion). *Lateral pterygoid:* draws the ipsilateral side of the mandible forward. *Acting bilaterally:* protraction of the jaw, a movement necessary for opening the mouth widely; lateral movement (producing grinding motion).

Palpation: Most patients with temporomandibular dysfunction suffer primarily from a muscular disorder that includes the involvement of the pterygoids. This muscle is rarely involved alone and is less likely to be tender than other masticatory muscles. The lateral pterygoid is one of the most commonly involved muscles in temporomandibular dysfunction. It is frequently overlooked as the source of the joint dysfunction.

Fibers of lateral pterygoid can be indirectly palpated through the masseter. Palpate with the mouth held open approximately 1 inch, or enough to relax the masseter sufficiently. Identify both the mandibular notch and the zygomatic process. Palpate just distal to the zygomatic process to identify tender areas of lateral pterygoid. It is frequently overlooked as the source of the joint dysfunction.

Palpate the upper fibers of medial pterygoid using a gloved finger inside the mouth. Slide the index finger lateral and posterior to the last molar. Identify the bony edge of the mandible. Move posteriorly and laterally to identify the medial pterygoid. Asking the patient to slowly bite down on a small object held between the teeth allows for clear identification of the contracting muscle.

Palpate the inferior fibers on the medial surface of the angle of the mandible. Allow the head to rotate slightly toward the side of the palpation to allow the neck muscles to soften. Reach up under the angle of the mandible approximately $3/8$ inch to identify the fibers of medial pterygoid.

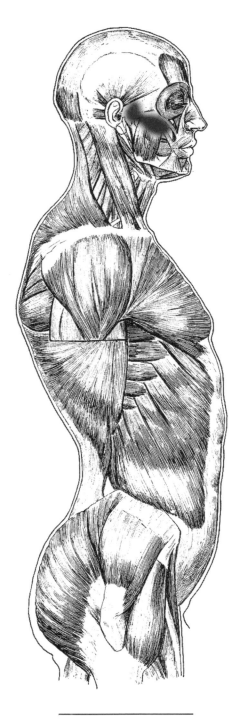

Lateral pterygoid pain pattern

Pain pattern: *Medial pterygoid:* Generalized pain in the mouth and the region of the temporomandibular joint—symptoms include throat soreness, difficulty swallowing, painful moderate restriction of jaw opening; lateral deviation of the incisal path, generally to the contralateral side; some limitation of full range of motion, possibly limiting the insertion of two stacked knuckles between the teeth. *Lateral pterygoid:* Pain in the region of the maxilla and the temporomandibular joint that might be associated with arthritis of the joint—symptoms such as temporomandibular joint disorders that include clicking of the jaw, restriction of the jaw opening, distortion of the incisal path, altered occlusion resulting in chewing dysfunction; excessive secretion off the maxillary sinus mimicking sinusitis; sometimes tinnitus. Note: Elimination of the zigzag of the incisal path when the tongue is placed on the posterior hard palate and the mouth is opened indicates pterygoid involvement.

Causative or perpetuating factors: *Medial pterygoid:* Forward head posture, bruxism, excessive gum chewing. Medial pterygoid is rarely involved alone and will be activated secondary to lateral pterygoid. *Lateral pterygoid:* As satellite trigger points to key trigger points in the neck muscles, especially the sternocleidomastoid; arthritis of the temporomandibular joint; bruxism; excessive gum chewing and nail biting; mandibular protrusion that might occur as when playing a wind instrument.

Satellite trigger points: *Medial pterygoid:* contralateral medial pterygoid, ipsilateral lateral pterygoid, masseter. *Lateral pterygoid:* contralateral medial and lateral pterygoid, masseter, ipsilateral temporalis.

Affected organ systems: Digestive system.

Associated zones, meridians, and points: Lateral zone; Foot Shao Yang Gall Bladder meridian, Foot Yang Ming Stomach meridian, Hand Tai Yang Small Intestine meridian; GB 2, ST 7, SI 18 and 19.

Stretch exercise: Ask the patient to slowly open the mouth against mild resistance placed on the lower jaw. Hold the jaw against light resistance for a count of three to five. Repeat three times. Following this stretch cycle, open and close the mouth several times without resistance. Note: This may be used as a trigger point release technique as well as stretch exercise for the patient.

Strengthening exercise: Due to the nature of this muscle, strengthening exercises are not necessary.

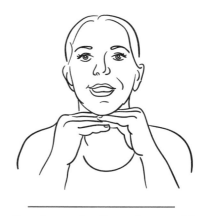

Stretch exercise: Lateral pterygoid

Muscles of the Shoulder Girdle

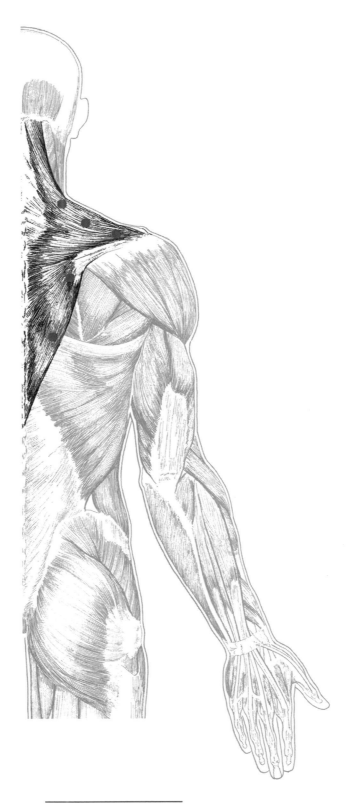

Trapezius and trigger points

Trapezius

Proximal attachment: External occipital protuberance, nuchal ligament, spinous processes of C1–T12.

Distal attachment: Spine of the scapula, acromion, lateral one-third of the clavicle.

Action: *Upper fibers:* flexion of the head and neck to the same side; elevation of the shoulder acting on the clavicle and the acromion. *Middle fibers:* retraction of the scapula. *Lower fibers:* depression of the scapula, rotation of the glenoid fossa upward.

Palpation: The trapezius is the muscle most commonly found to have constrictions and/or trigger point activity. To locate the trapezius, identify the following structures:

- Clavicle—Follow the curved course of the clavicle, from its articulation with the sternum to its articulation with the acromion. Medially the contours of the clavicle are convex; laterally its contours are concave.
- Spine of the scapula—Bony prominence of the upper scapula bounded laterally by the acromion, which forms the lateral tip of the shoulder girdle, and medially by the root of the spine of the scapula, the flattened, triangular surface located on a horizontal line with the spinous process of T3.
- External occipital protuberance—Locate the base of the skull at the midline, just superior to the cervical spinous processes. Moving superiorly from the midline onto the skull, you come to the external occipital protuberance. Its most prominent protrusion is called the inion, or the "bump of knowledge." Move laterally from the external occipital protuberance to palpate the superior nuchal lines, short transverse ridges that may or may not be palpable.
- Nuchal ligament—If the patient elongates his spine by pulling the crown of the head

up and dropping the chin in toward the throat, you will be able to palpate the cordlike nuchal ligament connecting the spinous processes of each of the cervical vertebrae. When the patient is relaxed the nuchal ligament will not be readily palpable.

- Spinous processes of C1–T12—Carefully differentiate each of the cervical and thoracic vertebrae, understanding that C1 spinous process cannot be palpated.

Begin by locating C7 and T1, the most prominent vertebrae at the base of the neck. With the patient seated, place the middle finger of one hand on the most prominent vertebra at the base of the neck. This is probably C7; however, it may be C6. To differentiate the two, place your index finger on the spinous process above your middle finger; place your ring finger on the spinous process distal to it. Ask the patient to extend his head. By doing so C6 will appear to move anteriorly under the palpating finger; C7 will remain fixed, as will T1.

Once C7 has been clearly noted, begin counting spinous processes of the cervical vertebrae superiorly until you reach the spinous process of C2; then count the spinous processes of the thoracic vertebrae distally until you reach T12.

To palpate the trapezius muscle, begin at the superior nuchal line and follow the muscle distally toward the angle of the neck. The contours of the upper fibers will take your hands anteriorly along the free edge of the trapezius to the lateral one-third of the clavicle. Palpate for the quality and consistency of the muscle between the lateral clavicle and the spine of the scapula, moving toward the root of the spine of the scapula. Continue the palpation of the muscle distally as it narrows to its characteristic triangular apex at T12.

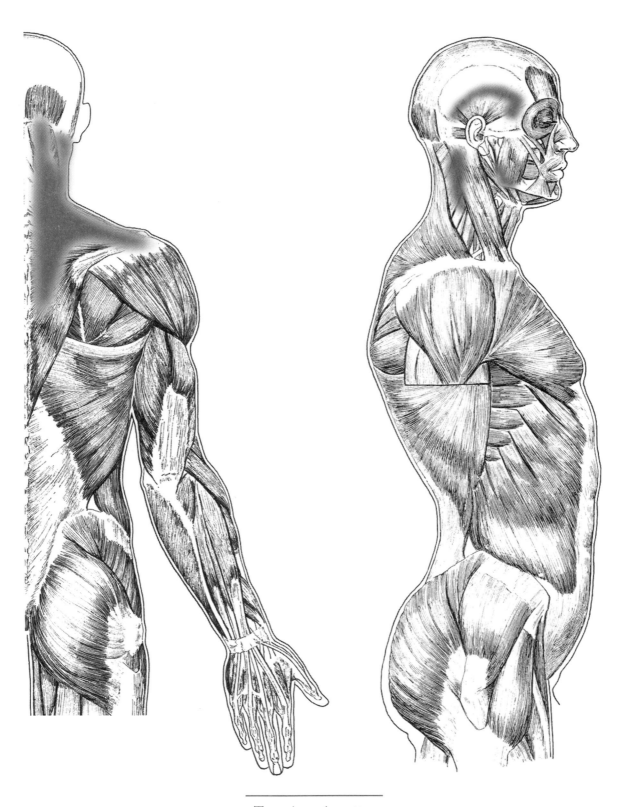

Trapezius pain pattern

Pain pattern: *Upper fibers:* upper trigger points cause pain along the posterolateral aspect of the neck, behind the ear and possibly to the temple. *Middle fibers:* intermediate trigger points cause pain toward the vertebrae, in the interscapular region and the lateral aspect of the posterior shoulder. *Lower fibers:* lower trigger points refer pain to the neck, suprascapular, and interscapular regions. Pain is accompanied by little restriction of motion.

Causative or perpetuating factors: Sustained lateral flexion of the head and neck and/or elevation of the shoulders; compression of the upper shoulders; whiplash trauma from the side.

Satellite trigger points: Supraspinatus, contralateral trapezius, levator scapulae.

Affected organ system: Respiratory system.

Associated zones, meridians, and points: Dorsal and lateral zones; Foot Tai Yang Bladder meridian (all yang meridians pass through the fibers of the upper trapezius); SI 12–15, GB 20 and 21, SJ 15, BL 41–49.

Stretch exercises:

1. *Upper trapezius:* Bend the head toward the unaffected side, pressing the head forward to lift the occiput. Lean the ear toward the homolateral shoulder. While holding this position, grasp the wrist of the arm on the affected side behind the back and pull slightly toward the side of the bend. The muscle on the affected side will receive the stretch.

2. *Middle and lower trapezius:* Sitting in a chair, bend forward, head dropped. Cross each arm over the body to grasp the opposite knee.

Strengthening exercise: Isometric against mild resistance, the face positioned forward.

1. Place the palm heel on the forehead for resistance. Press the head forward, into the resistance.
2. Place the palm heel of the right hand on the right temple. Press the head toward the right, into the resistance.
3. Place the palm heel of the left hand on the left temple. Press the head toward the left, into the resistance.
4. Clasp the hands behind the head just below the crown. Press the head and neck posteriorly, into the resistance.

Hold each position for a count of five.

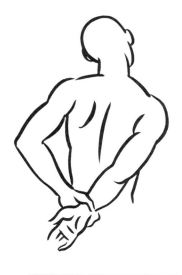

Stretch exercise 1: Trapezius

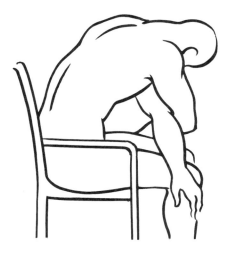

Stretch exercise 2: Trapezius

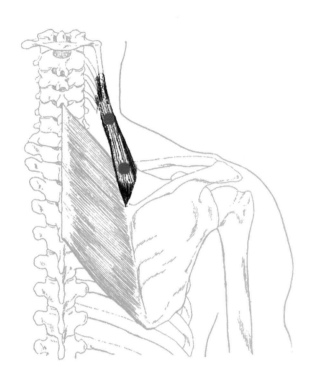

Levator scapulae and trigger points

LEVATOR SCAPULAE

Proximal attachment: Transverse processes of C1–C4.

Distal attachment: Medial aspect of the scapula from its superior angle to the root of the spine of the scapula.

Action: Elevation of the scapula. Assists in rotation of the neck to the same side; can assist in sidebending of the neck.

Palpation: The levator scapulae is second only to the trapezius in terms of the frequency with which it is beset by muscular constrictions and trigger point activity. The levator scapulae lies deep to the trapezius. As it moves from the superior aspect of the medial border of the scapula to the transverse processes of the cervical vertebrae, it becomes superficial at its middle one-third, which can be palpated directly at the angle of the neck (where the muscle lies between the trapezius and the sternocleidomastoid). Its distal one-third can be palpated through the trapezius when the trapezius is relaxed and when the levator scapulae harbors trigger points or is constricted. In order to differentiate this muscle from the overlying trapezius it is essential to pay strict attention to the direction of the muscle fibers. The fibers of the oblique levator scapulae run vertically and medially, deep to the fibers of the (also oblique) upper trapezius, which run laterally and horizontally.

To locate levator scapulae, identify the following structures:

- Root of the spine of the scapula—A small, triangular-shaped aspect of the scapula located at the medial border of the spine of the scapula. It most commonly lies on a horizontal line with T3.
- Transverse process of C1—Locate the angle of the mandible, the sharp lateral aspect of the jawbone. Moving posteriorly, the bony prominence of the transverse process of C1, lying between the angle of the mandible and the mastoid process, may be palpated on some people. Palpate bilaterally, gently, as this area may be quite tender.

To palpate the levator scapulae, place your patient in the prone position with his head resting comfortably in a face cradle. It is necessary for the head to be straight, not turned to one side or another, to successfully palpate this region. Your patient's arms should be at his sides with the palms up and the elbows slightly bent.

With your palpating hand, locate the angle of the scapula. Image the direction of the muscle fibers as they angle toward the upper cervical vertebrae. Using a cross-fiber technique, move superiorly back and forth over what you conceive the direction of fibers to be. Levator scapulae becomes superficial at the angle of the neck anterior to the free border of the trapezius.

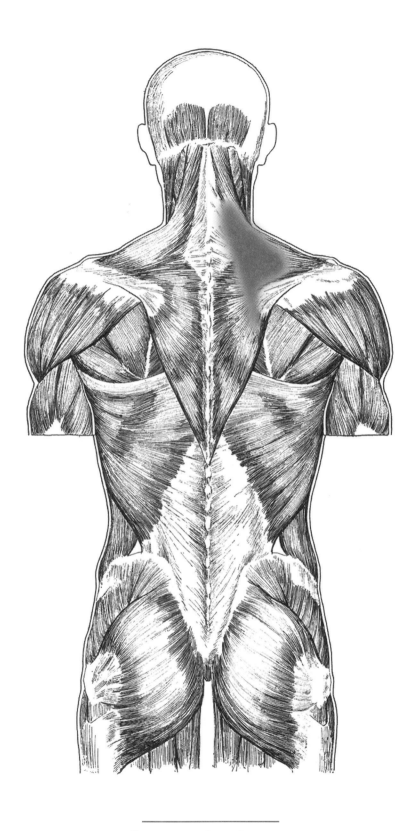

Levator scapulae pain pattern

Pain pattern: Pain at the angle of the neck and possibly at the posterior aspect of the shoulder and the midscapular region. There will be limited range of motion to the affected side.

Causative or perpetuating factors: Sustained rotation of the head and neck to one side; emotional tension; early stages of an acute upper respiratory infection.

Satellite trigger points: Splenius cervicis, scalenes, iliocostalis cervicis.

Affected organ system: Respiratory system.

Associated zones, meridians, and points: Dorsal zone; Foot Tai Yang Bladder meridian, Hand Tai Yang Small Intestine meridian; SI 13, 14, and 15.

Stretch exercises:

1. Bend the head toward the unaffected side, leaning the ear toward the homolateral shoulder. Rotate the face approximately 30 degrees to the unaffected side. Flex the neck slightly, directing the stretch forward and toward the unaffected side.
2. For a deeper stretch, while holding this position grasp the wrist of the arm on the affected side behind the back and pull slightly.

Strengthening exercise: Because the levator scapulae is a postural muscle, strengthening exercises are generally not necessary.

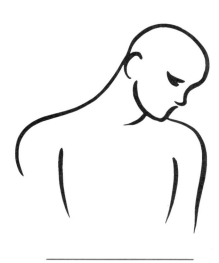

Stretch exercise 1: Levator scapulae

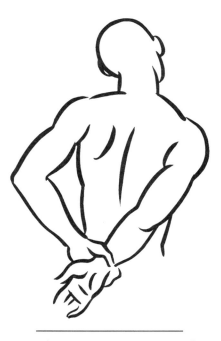

Stretch exercise 2: Levator scapulae

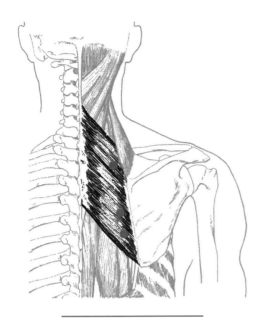

Rhomboids and trigger points

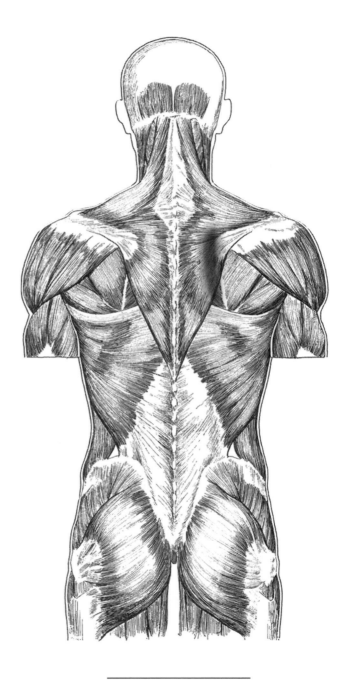

Rhomboids pain pattern

RHOMBOIDS

RHOMBOID MAJOR AND RHOMBOID MINOR

Proximal attachment: Spinous processes of C7–T5.

Distal attachment: Medial border of the scapula.

Action: Elevation and retraction of the scapula.

Palpation: To locate the rhomboids, identify the following structures:

- Medial border of the scapula
- Root of the spine of the scapula—A small, triangular-shaped aspect of the scapula located at the medial border of the spine of the scapula. It most commonly lies on a horizontal line with T3.
- Inferior angle of the scapula—The sharp, triangular, distal aspect of the scapula. In most cases the inferior angle of the scapula lies on a horizontal line with T7.
- Spinous processes of C7–T5

Position the patient prone on a treatment table with his face comfortably resting in a face cradle. Ask the patient to place his hand, palm up, at the small of his back. When he pushes posteriorly against resistance provided by your hand, the rhomboids become visible.

Palpate the rhomboids between the spinal column and the medial border of the scapula, through the fibers of the trapezius muscle.

Pain pattern: Pain concentrates along the medial border of the scapula but may spread laterally over the supraspinous area of the scapula. Local, superficial, aching pain is experienced at rest and is not influenced by movement.

Causative or perpetuating factors: Chronic overload due to prolonged periods working in a hunched-over position; postural overload due to an overly contracted pectoralis major.

Satellite trigger points: Levator scapulae, trapezius, infraspinatus, pectoralis major.

Affected organ system: Respiratory system.

Associated zones, meridians, and points: Dorsal zone; Foot Tai Yang Bladder meridian; BL 11–15, BL 41–44.

Stretch exercise: Sit in a chair. Bend forward, dropping the head. Cross each arm over the body to grasp the opposite knee. Hold this position for a count of five to ten.

Strengthening exercise: Lie diagonally across a bed or table, your arms hanging over the edge. Bend the elbows to 90 degrees. Retract the scapulae. Hold this position for a count of ten. Release and repeat.

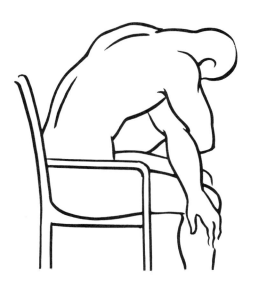

Stretch exercise: Rhomboids

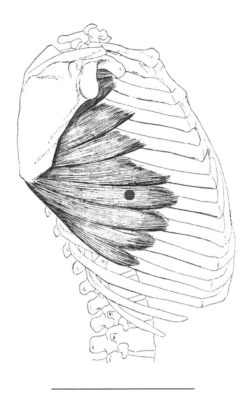

Serratus anterior and trigger point

SERRATUS ANTERIOR

Anterior attachment: Through slips (digitations) lying on the anterolateral aspect of rib 1 through ribs 8 or 9.

Posterior attachment: Passing deep to the scapula to attach to the costal surface of the full length of the scapula's medial border, with the heaviest attachment onto its inferior angle.

Action: Protraction of the scapula; lateral rotation of the scapula resulting in upward rotation of the glenoid fossa; assists in upward rotation and elevation of the scapula; stabilizes the scapula against the thoracic wall during forward-pushing movements.

Palpation: Serratus anterior, lying on the lateral aspect of the thoracic wall, forms the medial wall of the axilla. At its anterior attachment to the lower ribs, slips of this muscle interdigitate with the costal attachment of external oblique. Locate the serratus anterior with the patient lying on his side, the arm flexed and extended backward toward the surface of the table. Palpate superficially at the midaxillary line at the level of ribs 5 or 6, on the same horizontal line with the nipple. Palpate distally to ribs 8 and 9 to identify slips of the lower aspect of the serratus anterior; palpate superiorly from the midline to palpate slips of serratus anterior lying on ribs 1 through 5. Trigger points are most commonly found at the midaxillary line at the level of ribs 5 and 6. However, trigger points can develop in any of the slips (digitations) of serratus anterior.

Pain pattern: Pain in the anterolateral aspect of the chest as well as the medial to the inferior angle of the scapula. Pain may radiate down the ulnar surface of the homolateral arm and may extend as far as the palm and the ring finger. Symptoms include pain that is persistent, intense, and unaffected by movement or position; shortness of breath or the inability to take a deep breath without pain; inability to expand the lower chest during inspiration; breast or nipple pain.

Causative or perpetuating factors: Fast or prolonged running, push-ups, overhead lifting, chin-ups, severe coughing.

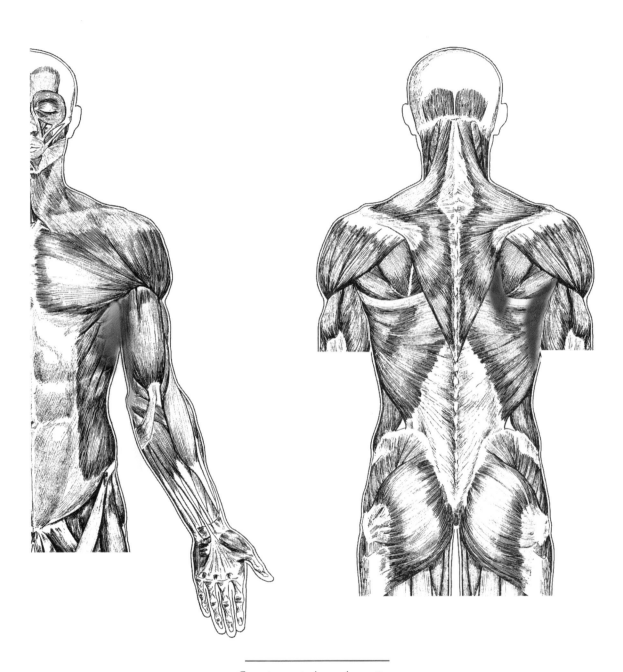

Serratus anterior pain pattern

Satellite trigger points: Latissimus dorsi, scalenes, and sternocleidomastoid (the accessory muscles of breathing).

Affected organ systems: Respiratory and digestive systems.

Associated zones, meridians, and points: Lateral zone; Hand Tai Yin Lung meridian, Foot Tai Yin Spleen meridian, Foot Shao Yang Gall Bladder meridian; SP 21, GB 22 and 23.

Stretch exercises:

1. Sitting on a chair, place the arm of the affected side over the back of the chair and hold the seat of the chair behind you. Using that arm to fix your shoulder blade, slowly turn your thorax in the opposite direction—for example, if the painful side is your left side, hold the back of the chair with your left arm and turn your torso toward the right.

2. Lower and middle positions of the doorway stretch—see page 81: With the forearms placed firmly on each side of a doorway, stretch the body through the outstretched arms, opening the chest and anterior shoulder region. Position 1: place the palms approximately at ear level. Position 2: place the elbows level with the shoulders.

Strengthening exercise: No strengthening exercise is needed due to the nature of this muscle.

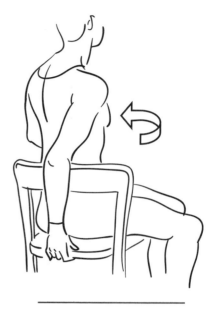

Stretch exercise: Serratus anterior

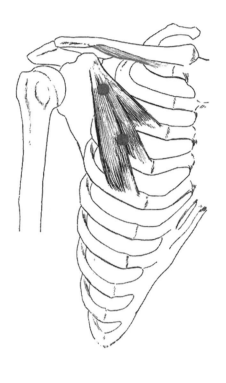

Pectoralis minor and trigger points

PECTORALIS MINOR

Proximal attachment: Coracoid process of the scapula.

Distal attachment: Anterior chest wall, on the upper surfaces of ribs 3, 4, and 5.

Action: Pulls the scapula and shoulder down and forward; assists in forced inspiration.

Palpation: Pectoralis minor lies deep to pectoralis major and may be difficult to palpate. During palpation the two pectoralis muscles may be differentiated by the direction of their fibers.

To locate pectoralis minor, identify the following structures:

• Coracoid process of the scapula—Projecting anteriorly from the superior border of the head of the scapula. Find the most concave aspect of the lateral clavicle; move your palpating hand distally approximately 1 inch into the deltopectoral triangle. Pressing posterolaterally, you will feel the coracoid process as a bony prominence. This area can be quite sensitive.

• Ribs 2 through 5—Locate the sternal articulations of ribs 2 through 5. Follow the course of each rib and rib space from the sternum toward the shoulder, noting the upward contours of the ribs as you palpate laterally. Note that rib 1 lies under the clavicle and so cannot be easily distinguished through palpation. Rib 2 is the first distinctly palpable rib distal to the clavicle.

Ask the patient to lie supine with his forearm resting comfortably on his body at the level of his waist. Ask him to bring his shoulder forward (anterior) by lifting his scapula off the table and then to take a deep breath. Palpation at the area of pectoralis minor will note the then-activated muscle. Palpate through pectoralis major to detect constricted fibers of pectoralis minor.

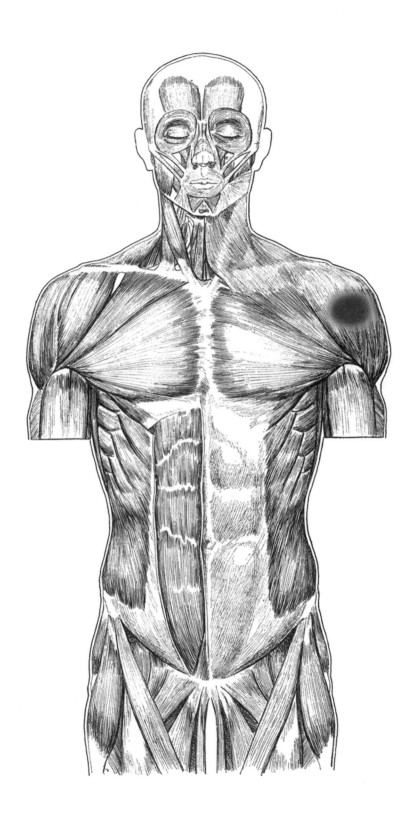

Pectoralis minor pain pattern

Pain pattern: Pain is referred to the front of the shoulder (anterior deltoid region) and possibly the front of the chest; some pain may be referred down the ulnar aspect of the arm to the fourth and fifth digits. Symptoms may include limitation in reaching forward and up or in reaching backward with the arm at the level of the shoulder.

Causative or perpetuating factors: Stooped, forward-leaning posture; compression, as that which might occur from the pressure of a backpack strap on the area.

Satellite trigger points: Pectoralis major, anterior deltoid, scalenes, sternocleidomastoid.

Affected organ system: Respiratory system.

Associated zones, meridians, and points: Ventral zone; Hand Tai Yin Lung meridian; SP 19 and 20.

Stretch exercise: With the forearms placed firmly on each side of a doorway, the palms approximately at ear level, stretch the body through the outstretched arms, opening the chest and anterior shoulder region. It is essential that the stretch is sufficient to retract the scapulae.

Strengthening exercise: Because the pectoralis minor is a postural muscle, strengthening exercises are generally not necessary.

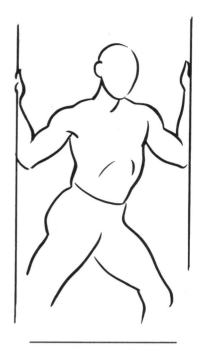

Stretch exercise: Pectoralis minor

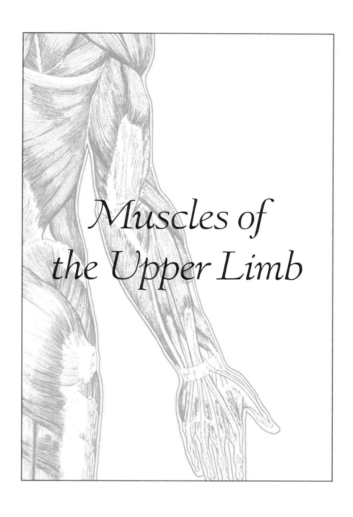

Muscles of
the Upper Limb

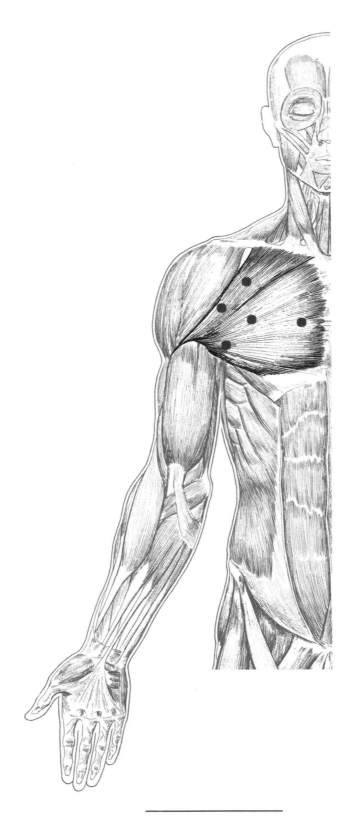

Pectoralis major and trigger points

PECTORALIS MAJOR

Proximal attachment: Medial two-thirds of the clavicle; sternum; costal cartilages of ribs 2–7; superficial aponeuroses of the external oblique and rectus abdominis.

Distal attachment: Lateral lip of the bicipital groove of the humerus.

Action: Adduction and medial rotation of the arm. *Clavicular fibers:* flexion of the arm, as in touching the lobe of the opposite ear.

Palpation: Pectoralis major forms the anterior wall of the axilla. As a superficial muscle of the chest wall, pectoralis major is clearly observable when the patient presses medially against his iliac crest.

To locate pectoralis major, identify the following structures:

- Clavicle—Follow the curved course of the clavicle, from its articulation with the sternum to its articulation with the acromion. Medially the contours of the clavicle are convex; laterally its contours are concave.
- Sternum—The breastbone: a long, flat bone that forms the center of the anterior thorax.
- Bicipital groove of the humerus (intertubercular groove)—Identify the greater and lesser tuberosities of the humerus, just distal to the lateral aspect of the acromion. (These are best palpated with the arm externally rotated.) The bicipital groove

lies medial to the greater tuberosity and lateral to the lesser tuberosity. Note that the tendon of the long head of the biceps brachii runs through the bicipital groove.

Locate pectoralis major with the patient lying supine, his arm resting at his side. Palpate pectoralis major throughout its course, beginning at its medial attachment at the sternum and the medial two-thirds of the distal aspect of the clavicle. Move laterally across the chest wall to its lateral attachment at the bicipital groove. The lateral aspect of the muscle, its free edge, may be lifted slightly off the chest wall in order to directly palpate the fibers using a pincer grasp palpation technique.

Pain pattern: Pain in the anterior aspect of the shoulder, at the anterior deltoid region; the pain pattern may include the anterior chest and breast. Pain may extend down the ulnar aspect of the arm to the fourth and fifth digits. Pain may sometimes mimic angina pectoris.

Causative or perpetuating factors: Overload stresses due to heavy lifting with arms in front of the body; immobilization of the arm in an adducted position; sustained round-shouldered position; sustained anxiety levels; referred phenomena via a viscerosomatic route associated with cardiac infarction.

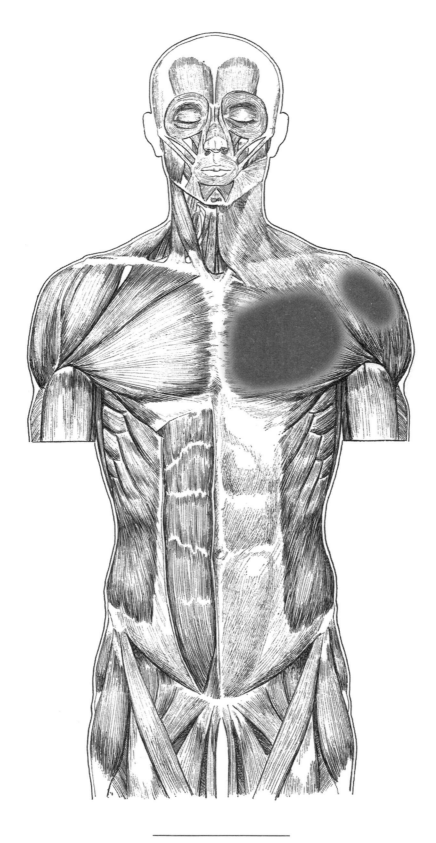

Pectoralis major pain pattern

Satellite trigger points: Anterior deltoid, sternocleidomastoid, scalenes, trapezius, rhomboids.

Affected organ systems: Respiratory and cardiovascular systems.

Associated zones, meridians, and points: Ventral zone; Foot Yang Ming Stomach meridian, Hand Tai Yin Lung meridian, Foot Tai Yin Spleen meridian, Foot Shao Yin Kidney meridian; ST 14, 15, and 16; ST 18; LU 1, 2, and 3; SP 19 and 20; KI 22–27.

Stretch exercise: With the forearms placed firmly on each side of a doorway, stretch the body through the outstretched arms, opening the chest and anterior shoulder region.

1. Place the palms approximately at ear level to stretch the upper fibers of pectoralis major.
2. Place the elbows level with the shoulders to stretch the middle fibers of pectoralis major.
3. Extend the arms fully, placing the hands well above the level of the head to stretch the lower fibers of pectoralis major.

Strengthening exercise: Lie in the supine position, arms abducted to 90 degrees and palms facing the ceiling. Horizontally flex the arms across the chest, keeping the elbows straight. Slowly return the arms to the starting position. Repeat five to ten times, flexing to a count of two and returning to the starting position to a count of four.

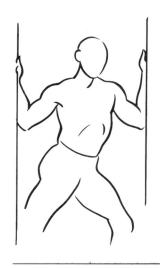

Stretch exercise 1: Pectoralis major

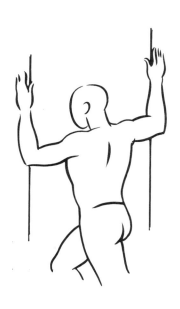

Stretch exercise 2: Pectoralis major

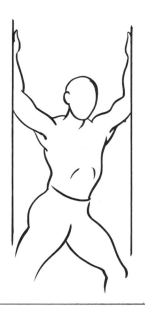

Stretch exercise 3: Pectoralis major

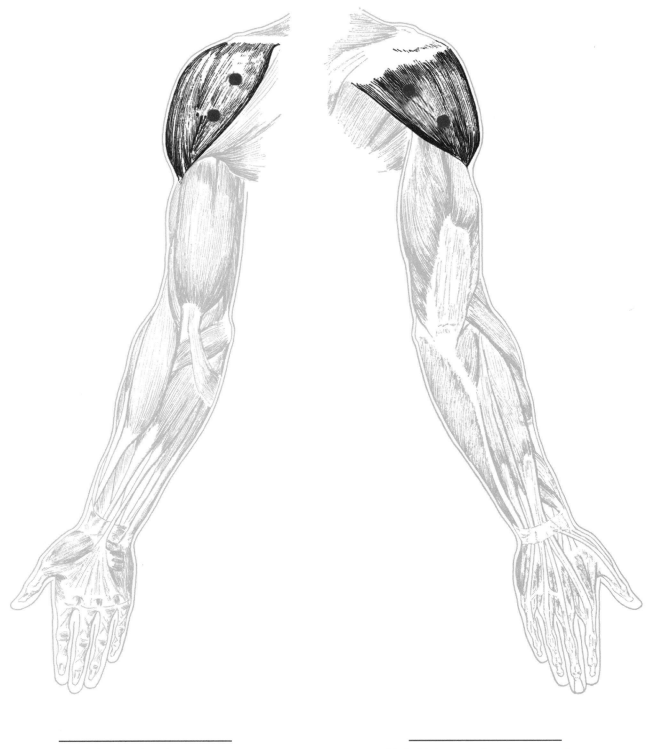

Deltoid (anterior) and trigger points

Deltoid (posterior) and trigger points

DELTOID

Proximal attachment: *Anterior fibers:* lateral one-third of the clavicle. *Medial fibers:* acromion. *Posterior fibers:* spine of the scapula.

Distal attachment: Deltoid tuberosity of the humerus.

Action: *Anterior fibers:* flexion and internal rotation of the humerus. *Medial fibers:* abduction of the humerus. *Posterior fibers:* extension and external rotation of the humerus.

Palpation: To locate the deltoid, identify the following structures:

- Clavicle—Follow the curved course of the clavicle, from its articulation with the sternum to its articulation with the acromion. Medially the contours of the clavicle are convex; laterally its contours are concave. The anterior deltoid attaches to the clavicle at its lateral concavity where the pectoralis major muscle ends.
- Acromion—The flat, lateral aspect of the scapula at the most lateral tip of the shoulder girdle. Abducting the humerus as you palpate the lateral tip of the shoulder girdle, you can clearly distinguish between the acromion and the head of the humerus.

- Spine of the scapula—Follow the course of the acromion posteriorly and medially along the spine of the scapula to the root of the spine of the scapula, a flattened, triangular surface at the medial border of the scapula. The root of the spine of the scapula is located on a horizontal line with the spinous process of T3.
- Deltoid tuberosity of the humerus—The bony prominence located approximately midway down the lateral aspect of the humerus.

Palpate the deltoid from its attachments on the shoulder girdle to its attachment on the humerus. Palpate anteriorly, noting the area where the deltoid lies adjacent to the pectoralis at the lateral concavity of the clavicle. Note the deltopectoral groove formed by the junction of the deltoid and pectoralis major muscles. Palpate the medial fibers, noting the attachment of the deltoid muscle to the acromion; palpate posteriorly, noting the attachment to the spine of the scapula. Note how the three aspects of the muscle converge to insert onto the deltoid tuberosity of the humerus.

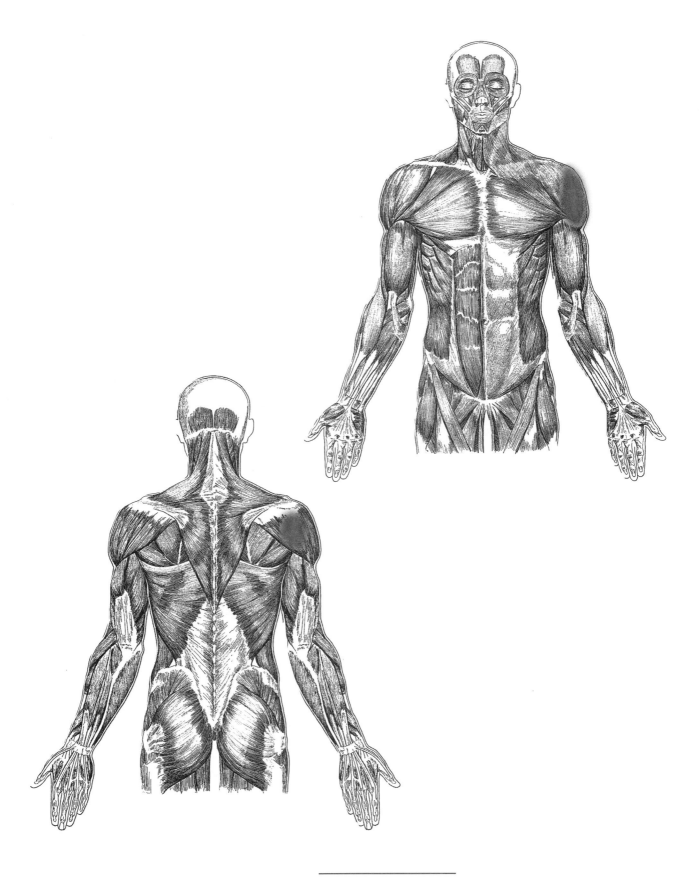

Deltoid pain pattern

Pain pattern: *Anterior fibers:* Pain is experienced in the anterior and medial deltoid; the patient may experience weakened abduction of the externally rotated arm. *Posterior fibers:* Pain is experienced in the posterior and medial deltoid; the patient may experience weakened abduction of the internally rotated arm.

Causative or perpetuating factors: Direct trauma due to impact, overexertion, or sudden overload.

Satellite trigger points: *Anterior fibers:* pectoralis major, biceps brachii, posterior deltoid. *Posterior fibers:* long head of the triceps, latissimus dorsi, teres major.

Affected organ systems: *Anterior fibers:* respiratory system. *Posterior fibers:* digestive system.

Associated zones, meridians, and points: *Anterior fibers:* ventral zone; Hand Tai Yin Lung meridian; LU 1, 2, and 3. *Posterior fibers:* dorsal and lateral zones; Hand Yang Ming Colon meridian, Hand Shao Yang Triple Warmer meridian; CO 14 and 15, SI 10; TW 13 and 14.

Stretch exercises:

1. *Anterior fibers:* Place the palms firmly on each side of a doorway at approximately ear level. Stretch the body through the outstretched arms, opening the chest and anterior shoulder region.

2. *Posterior fibers:* Pull the affected arm across the chest, using the other arm placed proximal to the elbow to guide the action.

Strengthening exercises: Both strengthening exercises should be performed in a standing position with the arms at the sides.

1. Flex the affected arms—keeping the elbows straight, bring the arm to shoulder level. Perform this flexion to a count of two; return to the starting position to a count of four. Repeat eight to ten times, increasing the number of repetitions as strength allows. Hand weights may be used to increase the work effort of the muscle.

2. Abduct the affected arm, keeping the elbows straight; bring the arm to shoulder level. Abduct to a count of two; return to the starting position to a count of four. Repeat eight to ten times, increasing the number of repetitions as strength allows. Hand weights may be used to increase the work effort of the muscle.

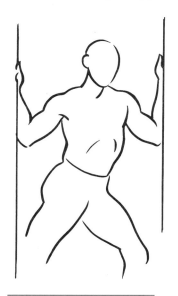

Stretch exercise 1: Anterior deltoid

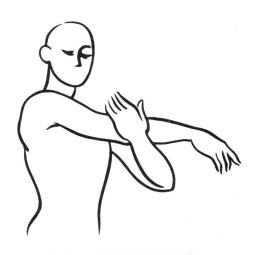

Stretch exercise 2: Posterior deltoid

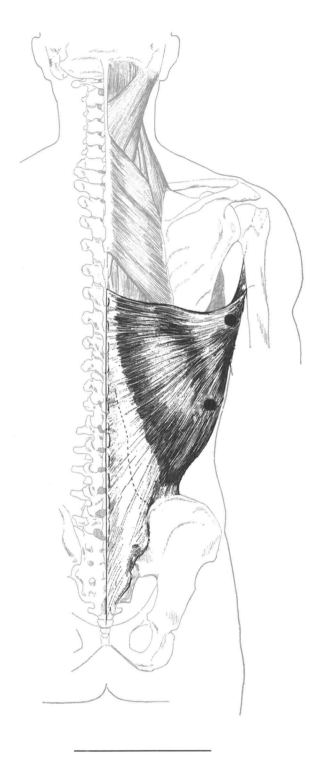

Latissimus dorsi and trigger points

LATISSIMUS DORSI

Proximal attachment: Latissimus dorsi fuses with teres major to attach at the medial edge of the bicipital groove, on the anterior aspect of the humerus.

Distal attachment: Spinous processes of T6–T12, L1–L5 and the sacrum, iliac crest via the thoracolumbar aponeurosis, lower 3–4 ribs, inferior angle of the scapula.

Action: Extension, adduction, and internal rotation of the arm at the shoulder.

Palpation: The latissimus dorsi and the teres major together form the posterior wall of the axilla. The tendon of the latissimus dorsi twists upon itself before fusing with teres major at the attachment on the bicipital groove.

To locate latissimus dorsi, identify the following structures:

- Spinous processes of T6 through T12 and L1 through L5—Note the difference in the size and shape of the spinous processes of the thoracic vertebrae versus the lumbar vertebrae.
- Iliac crests—Lying on a horizontal line with the junction of L4–L5.

- Inferior angle of the scapula—The sharp, triangular, distal aspect of the scapula. In most cases the inferior angle of the scapula lies on a horizontal line with T7.
- Bicipital groove of the humerus (intertubercular groove)—Identify the greater and lesser tuberosities of the humerus, just distal to the lateral aspect of the acromion. (These are best palpated with the arm externally rotated.) The bicipital groove lies medial to the greater tuberosity and lateral to the lesser tuberosity. Note that the tendon of the long head of the biceps brachii runs through the bicipital groove.

Palpate latissimus dorsi with the patient in the prone position, arms resting at his sides, palms up. Use a pincer grasp at the posterior axillary fold, gently lifting the muscle off the thoracic wall. Grasp the muscle along its lateral placement, proximal to the inferior angle of the scapula, at approximately the midpoint of the lateral edge of the scapula; follow the muscle toward the iliac crest, where the muscle fibers become increasingly indistinct.

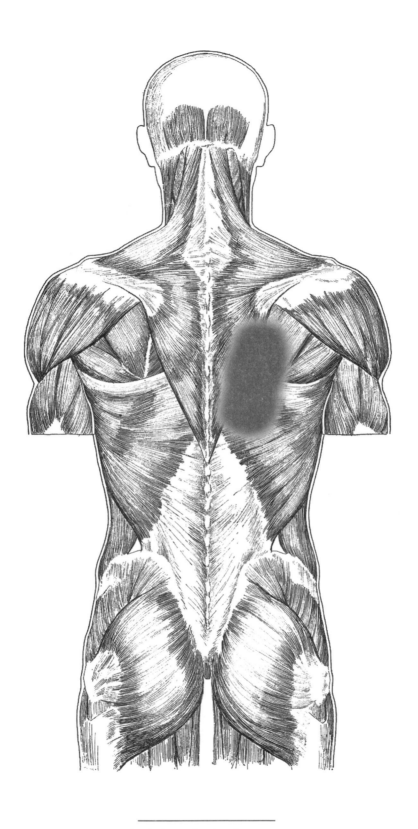

Latissimus dorsi pain pattern

Pain pattern: Pain is located at the inferior angle of the scapula and the surrounding midthoracic region, possibly extending to the back of the shoulder and down the medial aspect of the arm, forearm, and hand, including the ring and little fingers. The nature of the pain is an ache that shows neither aggravation nor relief with activity or change of position.

Causative or perpetuating factors: Depressor movements that overload, as in pulling something down from above or holding a heavy, bulky object.

Satellite trigger points: Teres major, triceps brachii, rectus abdominis, iliocostalis thoracis, and iliocostalis lumborum.

Affected organ system: Digestive system.

Associated zones, meridians, and points: Dorsal and lateral zones; Foot Tai Yang Bladder meridian, Hand Tai Yang Small Intestine meridian; BL 23, SI 9.

Stretch exercise: Reach both arms above the head. Grasp the wrist of the hand on the affected side with the opposite hand. Pull the wrist and arm toward the unaffected side, bending the torso to that side. Hold this position for a count of ten to fifteen.

Strengthening exercise: Standing with the legs shoulder-width apart, bend from the waist so that the upper body is parallel to the floor. Reach the arm of the affected side toward the opposite foot. Bend the elbow to make a 90-degree angle and retract the scapula, extending the upper arm, bringing it to a position alongside the torso. The final position is one in which both the torso and the upper arm are parallel to the floor while the forearm is perpendicular to the floor. Draw the arm to the side to a count of two. Reach for the opposite foot to a count of four.

Repeat eight to ten times, increasing repetitions as the strength of the muscle allows. Do not allow the torso to move during the course of the exercise.

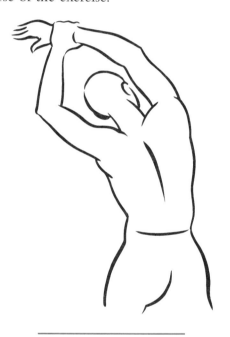

Stretch exercise: Latissimus dorsi

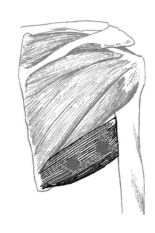

Teres major and trigger points

TERES MAJOR

Proximal attachment: Teres major fuses with latissimus dorsi to attach at the medial edge of the bicipital groove, on the anterior aspect of the humerus.

Distal attachment: Inferior angle of the scapula.

Action: Internal rotation, adduction, and extension of the arm.

Palpation: Teres major and latissimus dorsi are fused at their insertion into the bicipital groove. The tendon of latissimus dorsi twists upon itself before fusing with teres major at the attachment at the bicipital groove.

To locate teres major, identify the following structures:

• Inferior angle of the scapula—The sharp, triangular, distal aspect of the scapula. In most cases the inferior angle of the scapula lies on a horizontal line with T7.

• Bicipital groove of the humerus (intertubercular groove)—Identify the greater and lesser tuberosities of the humerus, just distal to the lateral aspect of the acromion. (These are best palpated with the arm externally rotated.) The bicipital groove lies medial to the greater tuberosity and lateral to the lesser tuberosity. Note that the tendon of the long head of the biceps brachii runs through the bicipital groove.

Palpate teres major at the posterior axillary fold, deeper and more medial than latissimus dorsi. Taut bands or trigger points within teres major will be found proximal to the midpoint of the lateral edge of the scapula.

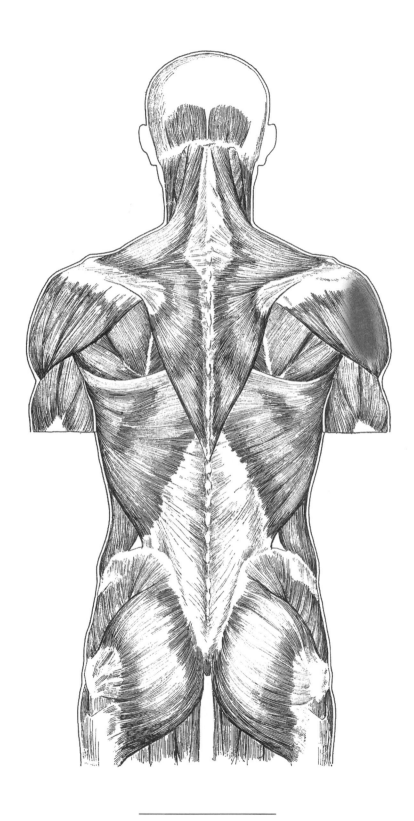

Teres major pain pattern

Pain pattern: Pain is referred to the posterior deltoid region. Pain may extend to the extensor surface of the forearm. Patient has difficulty abducting the arm and placing it against the homolateral ear. Pain is experienced when reaching forward and up, and there is little restriction of motion.

Causative or perpetuating factors: Depressor movements that overload, as in pulling something down from above or holding a heavy, bulky object.

Satellite trigger points: Long head of the triceps brachii, latissimus dorsi, posterior deltoid, teres minor, subscapularis.

Affected organ system: Digestive system.

Associated zones, meridians, and points: Dorsal zone; Hand Tai Yang Small Intestine meridian; SI 9.

Stretch exercises:

1. Reach both arms above the head. Grasp the wrist of the hand on the affected side with the opposite hand. Pull the wrist and arm toward the unaffected side, bending the torso to that side. Hold this position for a count of ten to fifteen.

2. Stand, or lie supine, with the elbow of the affected side close to the ear, forearm behind the head. Pull the elbow toward the opposite side.

Strengthening exercise: Standing with the legs shoulder-width apart, bend from the waist so the upper body is parallel to the floor. Reach the arm of the affected side toward the opposite foot. Bend the elbow to make a 90-degree angle and retract the scapula, extending the upper arm, bringing it to a position alongside the torso. The final position is one in which both the torso and the upper arm are parallel to the floor, while the

forearm is perpendicular to the floor. Draw the arm to the side to a count of two. Reach for the opposite foot to a count of four.

Repeat eight to ten times, increasing repetitions as the strength of the muscle allows. Do not allow the torso to move during the course of the exercise.

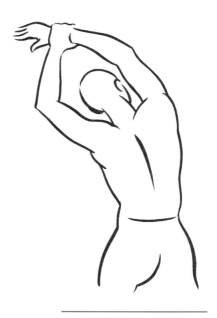

Stretch exercise 1: Teres major

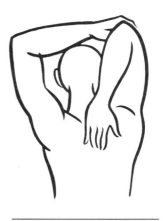

Stretch exercise 2: Teres major

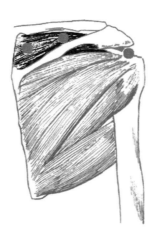

Supraspinatus and trigger points

Supraspinatus

Proximal attachment: Supraspinatus fossa of the scapula.

Distal attachment: Upper part of the greater tubercle of the humerus.

Action: Assists the deltoid in abduction of the humerus by pulling the head of the humerus inward toward the glenoid fossa. Aids in stabilizing the head of the humerus in the glenoid fossa.

Palpation: Supraspinatus is one of the four muscles that comprise the rotator cuff. The other muscles of the rotator cuff are infraspinatus, teres minor, and subscapularis. Supraspinatus lies deep to the trapezius.

To locate supraspinatus, identify the following structures:

- Supraspinatus fossa of the scapula—The dorsal aspect of the scapula lying proximal to the spine of the scapula.
- Acromion—The flat, lateral aspect of the scapula at the most lateral tip of the shoulder girdle. Abducting the humerus as you palpate the lateral tip of the shoulder girdle, you can clearly distinguish between the rectangular acromion and the head of the humerus.

To palpate supraspinatus, palpate deep to the trapezius in the supraspinatus fossa, moving laterally toward the acromion. Trigger points and areas of constriction most commonly can be palpated approximately 1 inch lateral to the medial (vertebral) border of the scapula just superior to the spine of the scapula and just medial to the acromion, between the clavicle and the spine of the scapula. Deep palpation is required to feel through the trapezius muscle; however, care should be taken to avoid forcing through constricted muscle in an effort to reach an underlying muscle.

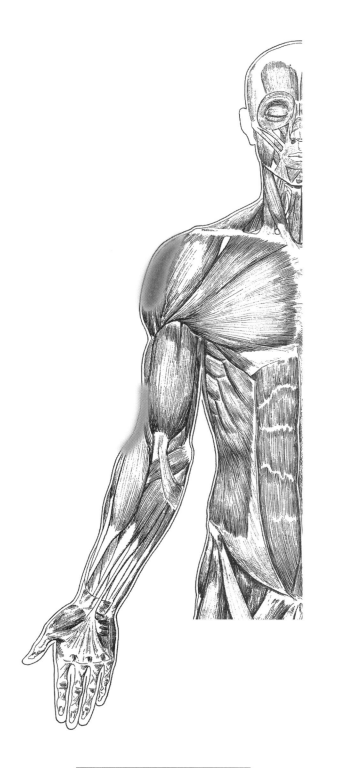

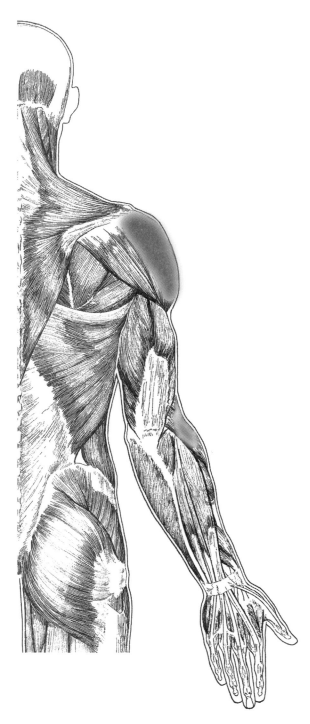

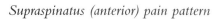

Supraspinatus (anterior) pain pattern

Supraspinatus (posterior) pain pattern

Pain pattern: Pain concentrates in the middle deltoid region and is experienced as a deep ache when the arm is at rest. The ache extends downward over the arm and forearm and sometimes focuses over the lateral epicondyle. Pain is commonly felt during abduction.

Causative or perpetuating factors: Carrying heavy objects with the arm hanging at the side.

Satellite trigger points: Subscapularis, infraspinatus, middle trapezius, upper trapezius, deltoid, latissimus dorsi.

Affected organ systems: Respiratory and digestive systems.

Associated zones, meridians, and points: Dorsal zone; Hand Yang Ming Colon meridian, Hand Tai Yang Small Intestine meridian, Hand Shao Yang Triple Warmer meridian; CO 16, SI 12, TW 14 and 15.

Stretch exercises:
1. Using the unaffected arm, pull the affected arm across the back at the level of the waist and pull up slightly. Hold this position for a count of fifteen to twenty.
2. As flexibility increases, reach the fingers of the affected arm toward the inferior angle of the opposite shoulder. Hold for a count of fifteen to twenty.

Strengthening exercise: Abduct the arms, keeping the elbows straight. Abduct to a count of two; return to the starting position to a count of four. Repeat eight to ten times, increasing the number of repetitions as strength allows. Hand weights may be used to increase the work effort of the muscle. Supraspinatus will work in the first 15 to 20 degrees of abduction, before deltoid fully activates.

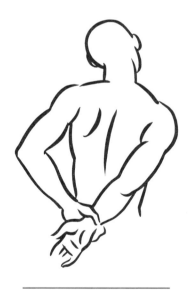

Stretch exercise 1: Supraspinatus

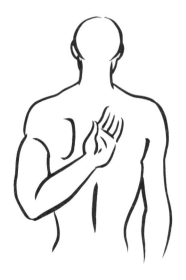

Stretch exercise 2: Supraspinatus

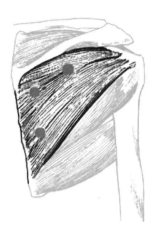

Infraspinatus and trigger points

INFRASPINATUS

Proximal attachment: Medial two-thirds of the infraspinatus fossa, which lies distal to the spine of the scapula.

Distal attachment: Posterior aspect of the greater tuberosity of the humerus, distal to the attachment of supraspinatus.

Action: External rotation of the arm; aids in stabilizing the head of the humerus in the glenoid fossa during upward movement of the arm, assisted by teres minor.

Palpation: Infraspinatus is one of the four muscles that comprise the rotator cuff. The other muscles of the rotator cuff are supraspinatus, teres minor, and subscapularis. Constrictions and trigger point activity in infraspinatus is one of the most common causes of shoulder pain. It is third only to upper trapezius and levator scapulae in frequency of involvement in trigger point activity.

To locate infraspinatus, identify the following structures:

- Infraspinatus fossa of the scapula—The aspect of the scapula that lies distal to the spine of the scapula.
- Greater tuberosity of the humerus—Distal to the lateral aspect of the acromion, easiest palpated when the arm is in external rotation. Differentiate the greater tuberosity from the lesser tuberosity, and locate the bicipital groove, which lies between them.

To palpate infraspinatus use flat digital palpation within the infraspinatus fossa, beginning at the medial (vertebral) border of the scapula and moving laterally toward the insertion at the greater tuberosity of the humerus. Constrictions and trigger points are most commonly found approximately $^1/_2$ to 1 inch distal to the spine of the scapula.

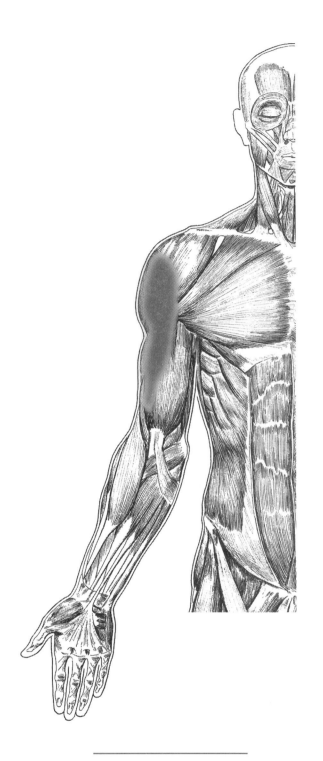

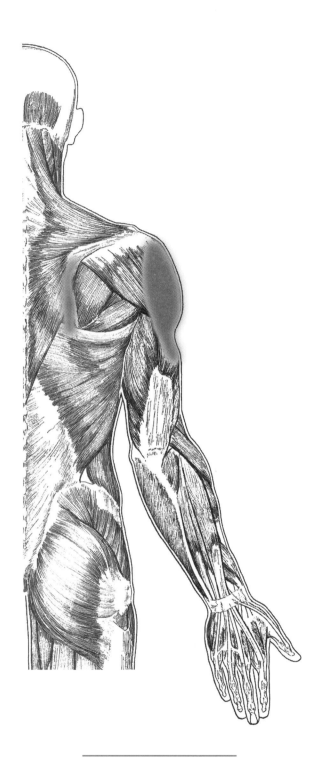

Infraspinatus (anterior) pain pattern

Infraspinatus (posterior) pain pattern

Pain pattern: Proximal trigger points refer pain deep in the anterior deltoid region and the shoulder joint, extending down the front and lateral aspects of the arm and possibly the forearm and the radial half of the hand. Pain may extend to the suboccipital region and posterior cervical areas. Distal trigger points refer pain between the spine of the scapula and the vertebral border of the scapula. Pain is experienced when sleeping on either side. The patient may be unable to reach behind his back.

Causative or perpetuating factors: Overload stresses while reaching backward and upward.

Satellite trigger points: Teres minor, anterior deltoid, posterior deltoid, biceps brachii, supraspinatus, teres major, latissimus dorsi.

Affected organ system: Digestive system.

Associated zones, meridians, and points: Dorsal zone; Hand Tai Yang Small Intestine meridian; SI 9, 10, and 11.

Stretch exercises:

1. Starting with the affected arm at 90 degrees horizontal abduction, extend the arm toward the back, internally rotating at the shoulder. At the limitation of extension, bend the elbow and touch the inferior angle of the opposite scapula.

2. Pull the affected arm across the chest, using the other arm placed proximal to the elbow to guide the action.

Strengthening exercise: Lie supine with the arm close to the torso and the elbow flexed to 90 degrees. Without moving the elbow and arm away from the torso, rotate the forearm as if to place the back of the hand on the floor. Return to the starting position.

Repeat eight to ten times. Hand weights may be used as strength develops, to increase the work effort placed on the muscle.

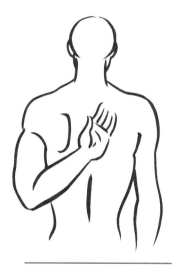

Stretch exercise 1: Infraspinatus

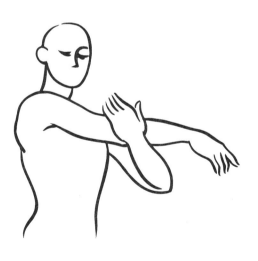

Stretch exercise 2: Infraspinatus

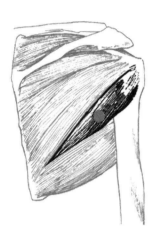

Teres minor and trigger point

TERES MINOR

Proximal attachment: Proximal two-thirds of the lateral border of the scapula, on the dorsal surface.

Distal attachment: Posterior aspect of the greater tuberosity of the humerus, distal to the attachment of infraspinatus.

Action: External rotation of the arm at the shoulder; acts with the infraspinatus to stabilize the head of the humerus during movement of the arm.

Palpation: Teres minor is one of the four muscles that comprise the rotator cuff. The other muscles of the rotator cuff are supraspinatus, infraspinatus, and subscapularis.

To locate teres minor, identify the following structures:

- Infraspinatus muscle—See muscle description on page 99.

- Teres major muscle—See muscle description on page 91.
- Greater tuberosity of the humerus—Distal to the lateral aspect of the acromion, easiest palpated when the arm is in external rotation. Differentiate the greater tuberosity from the lesser tuberosity, and locate the bicipital groove, which lies between them.

To palpate constrictions within teres minor, palpate near the lateral edge of the scapula between the infraspinatus, lying above teres minor, and teres major, lying below teres minor. Note that teres minor attaches on the posterior aspect of the humerus while teres major attaches on the anterior aspect of the humerus.

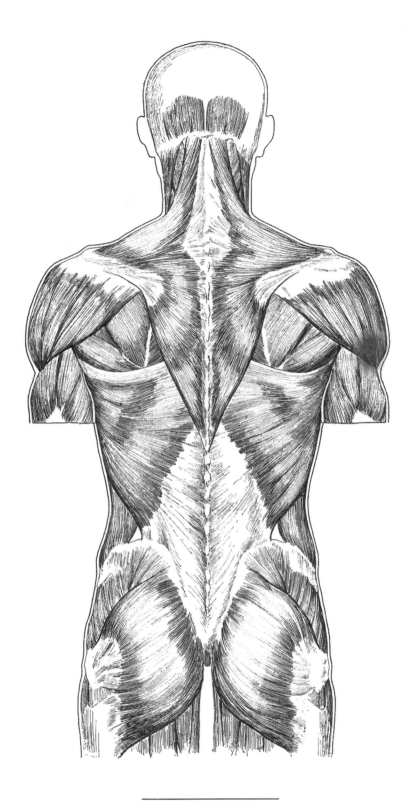

Teres minor pain pattern

Pain pattern: Pain in the distal posterior deltoid, possibly into the posterolateral upper arm. Pain may be sharply localized and deep in nature, and it becomes more apparent when pain and restrictions in infraspinatus are reduced. There is usually little restriction of movement.

Causative or perpetuating factors: Overload stresses when reaching backward and upward.

Satellite trigger points: Infraspinatus.

Affected organ system: Digestive system.

Associated zones, meridians, and points: Dorsal zone; Hand Tai Yang Small Intestine meridian; SI 9.

Stretch exercises:

1. Starting with the arm at 90 degrees horizontal abduction, extend the arm toward the back, internally rotating at the shoulder. At the limit of extension, bend the elbow and touch the inferior angle of the opposite scapula.

2. Pull the affected arm across the chest, using the other arm placed proximal to the elbow to guide the action.

Strengthening exercise: Lie supine with the arm close to the torso and the elbow flexed to 90 degrees. Without moving the elbow and arm away from the torso, rotate the forearm as if to place the back of the hand on the floor. Return to the starting position.

Repeat eight to ten times. Hand weights may be used as strength develops to increase the work effort placed on the muscle.

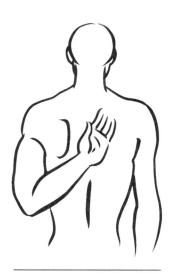

Stretch exercise 1: Teres minor

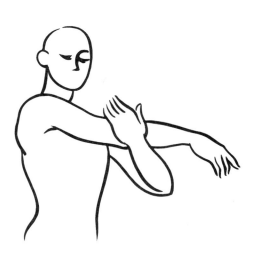

Stretch exercise 2: Teres minor

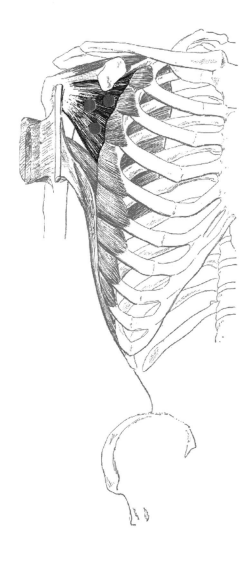

Subscapularis and trigger points

SUBSCAPULARIS

Proximal attachment: The subscapular fossa on the anterior (costal) surface of the scapula.

Distal attachment: Lesser tubercle of the humerus on the anterior aspect of the humerus.

Action: Internal rotation and adduction of the arm at the shoulder. Aids in stabilizing the head of the humerus in the glenoid fossa during movement of the arm.

Palpation: Subscapularis is one of the four muscles that comprise the rotator cuff. The other muscles of the rotator cuff are supraspinatus, infraspinatus, and teres minor. This muscle may be quite difficult to palpate given its location on the anterior aspect of the scapula, adjacent to the thorax.

To locate subscapularis, identify the following structures:

- Lateral border of the scapula
- Posterior wall of the axilla, formed by latissimus dorsi

Palpation of subscapularis can be accomplished with the patient in either the supine or prone position. To palpate subscapularis, abduct the arm. Using flat palpation, reach under (anterior to) the posterior axillary fold, moving medial to both latissimus dorsi and teres major. Feel for the hard lateral border of the scapula with the pads of the fingers. Continue to reach medially, palpating subscapularis against the anterior aspect of the scapula along its lateral border. The extent to which the muscle can be palpated will depend on the degree of flexibility of the patient's scapula on the thorax.

Pain pattern: Pain concentrates in the posterior deltoid area and may extend over the scapula and down the posterior aspect of the arm. It may skip the forearm to reappear as a band around the wrist. Symptoms are painful restriction of abduction and external rotation of the arm. Trigger points may contribute to a subluxation of the head of the humerus.

Causative or perpetuating factors: Repetitive exertion requiring internal rotation, as in the swimmer's crawl; sudden shoulder trauma.

Satellite trigger points: Pectoralis major, teres major, latissimus dorsi, long head of the triceps brachii, anterior deltoid, posterior deltoid.

Affected organ system: Respiratory system.

Associated zones, meridians, and points: Dorsal zone; Hand Tai Yang Small Intestine meridian; SI 9 and 10.

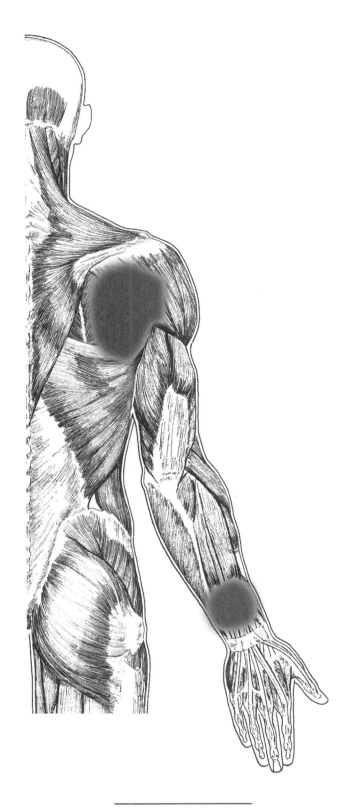

Subscapularis pain pattern

Stretch exercises:

1. Bend at the waist and rest one arm on a table, torso parallel to the floor. Allow the affected arm to hang straight down while holding a heavy weight. Move the weighted arm in small circles. This technique is also used to aid in the readjustment of the shoulder joint.

2. With the forearms placed firmly on each side of a doorway, stretch the body through the outstretched arms, opening the chest and anterior shoulder region. First perform the exercise with the elbows level with the shoulders. Then extend the arms fully, placing the hands well above the head.

3. With the elbow bent to 90 degrees, abduct the affected arm, raising the elbow to the shoulder level. Draw the forearm back behind the head. The stretch can be increased by applying a slight posterior pressure to the upper arm, just proximal to the elbow.

Strengthening exercise: Lie supine with the arm close to the torso and the elbow flexed to 90 degrees. Without moving the elbow and arm away from the torso, rotate the forearm as if to place the back of the hand on the floor. Return to the starting position.

Repeat eight to ten times. Hand weights may be used as strength develops to increase the work effort placed on the muscle.

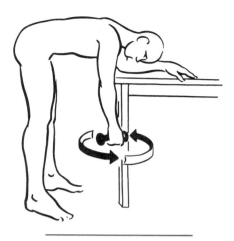

Stretch exercise 1: Subscapularis

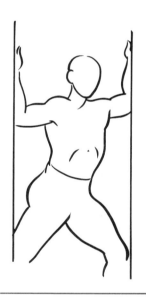

Stretch exercise 2: Subscapularis

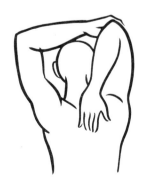

Stretch exercise 3: Subscapularis

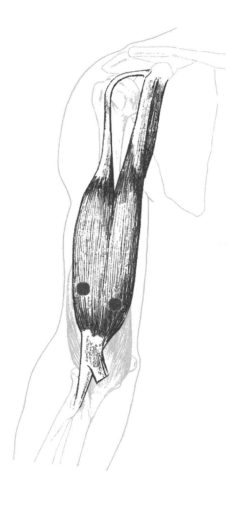

Biceps brachii and trigger points

BICEPS BRACHII

Proximal attachment: *Long head:* supraglenoid tubercle of the scapula. *Short head:* coracoid process of the scapula.

Distal attachment: Tuberosity of the radius.

Action: Flexion of the forearm at the elbow; assists in flexion of the arm at the shoulder. Aids in supination of the forearm against resistance when the elbow is flexed.

Palpation: To locate biceps brachii, identify the following structures:

- Bicipital groove of the humerus (intertubercular groove)—Identify the greater and lesser tuberosities of the humerus, just distal to the lateral aspect of the acromion. (These are best palpated with the arm externally rotated.) The bicipital groove lies medial to the greater tuberosity and lateral to the lesser tuberosity. Note that the tendon of the long head of the biceps brachii runs through the bicipital groove.

- Coracoid process of the scapula— Projecting anteriorly from the superior border of the head of the scapula. Find the most concave aspect of the lateral clavicle; move your palpating hand distally approximately 1 inch into the deltopectoral triangle. Pressing posterolaterally, you will feel the bony prominence of the coracoid process. This area can be quite sensitive.

The powerful biceps brachii can be palpated throughout its course. Flex the arm 15 to 45 degrees to locate the tendon of attachment on the (bicipital) tuberosity of the radius. Palpate biceps brachii, moving superiorly. The long head can be palpated by following its tendon of attachment as it passes through the bicipital groove. External rotation of the arm facilitates the ability to palpate the tendon within its groove. The short head can be palpated as it moves medially toward its attachment at the coracoid process of the scapula.

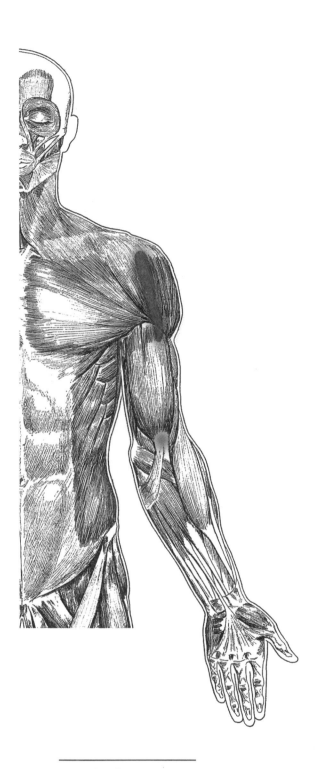

Biceps brachii pain pattern

Pain pattern: Superficial aching pain in the anterior shoulder and arm, with some restriction of motion.

Causative or perpetuating factors: Sustained elbow flexion; chronic or acute strain caused by sports or heavy lifting.

Satellite trigger points: Brachialis, supinator, triceps brachii.

Affected organ system: Respiratory system.

Associated zones, meridians, and points: Ventral zone; Hand Tai Yin Lung meridian, Hand Jue Yin Pericardium meridian; LU 3,4, and 5; PC 2 and 3.

Stretch exercise: Hold on to a doorjamb with the affected arm. The hand should be at shoulder level with the elbow straight and the thumb pointing toward the floor. Turn the body away from the arm without allowing any joint to bend. Hold this position for a count of fifteen to twenty.

Strengthening exercise: Stand with the arms at your sides, palms facing toward the body. Flex the forearms and, keeping the elbows close to the body, draw the palms toward the shoulder. Slowly return to the starting position. Flex to a count of two; release to a count of four.

Now stand with the arms at your sides, this time with palms facing outward. Flex the forearms and, keeping the elbows close to the body, draw the palms toward the shoulder. Slowly return to the starting position. Flex to a count of two; release to a count of four.

Repeat both exercises eight to ten times, increasing repetitions as strength allows. Hand weights may be used to increase the work effort placed on the muscle.

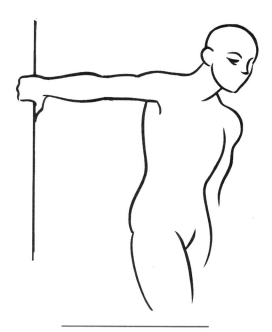

Stretch exercise: Biceps brachii

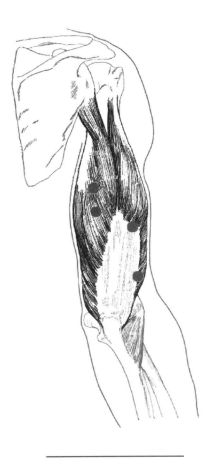

Triceps brachii and trigger points

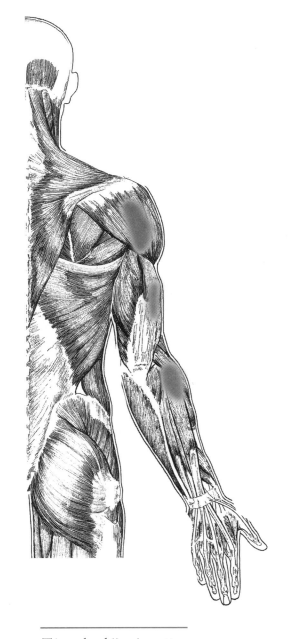

Triceps brachii pain pattern

Triceps Brachii

Proximal attachment: *Long head:* infraglenoid lip of the scapula. *Lateral head:* posterior humerus, superior to the radial groove. *Medial head:* posterior humerus, inferior to the radial groove.

Distal attachment: Via a common tendon to the olecranon process of the ulna.

Action: Extension of the forearm at the elbow. *Long head:* aids in extension and adduction of the arm at the shoulder.

Palpation: To locate triceps brachii, identify the following structures:

- Head of the humerus
- Olecranon process of the ulna—Large process at the proximal end of the ulna

Palpate the triceps muscle throughout its course, moving from the olecranon process proximally along the posterior humerus. Palpate the long head to its attachment on the scapula, then return to the body of the muscle where it forms a common muscular belly with the lateral head. The medial head lies deep to the long head, but it can be palpated at the distal aspect of the medial humerus. Palpate both the posterolateral and the posteromedial aspects of the arm for taut bands and areas of constriction within the body of the muscle.

Pain pattern: Pain throughout the posterior aspect of the arm, including the lateral epicondyle. Pain may be experienced in the fourth and fifth digits and/or the suprascapular region. If constrictions or trigger points are located in the long head, the patient may be unable to straighten his arm against his ear while holding the arm up above his head.

Causative or perpetuating factors: Overload stresses associated with pushing heavy objects or with rapid extension of the forearm.

Satellite trigger points: Latissimus dorsi, teres major, teres minor, anconeus, supinator, brachioradialis, extensor carpi radialis.

Affected organ system: Digestive system.

Associated zones, meridians, and points: Dorsal zone; Hand Shao Yang Triple Warmer meridian; TW 10–13.

Stretch exercise: Place the palm of the hand of the affected arm on the spine of the homolateral scapula. Draw the elbow toward the ear and back behind the head. Gentle posterior pressure to the region proximal to the elbow will increase the stretch. Hold this position for a count of ten to fifteen.

Strengthening exercise: Stand or sit in a comfortable position. Place the hand near the spine of the homolateral scapula, drawing the elbow toward the ear. Without moving the upper arm, extend the elbow, straightening the arm. Extend to a count of two; return to the starting position to a count of four.

Repeat eight to ten times, increasing repetitions as strength of the muscle allows. Hand weights may be used to increase the work effort of the muscle.

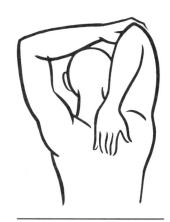

Stretch exercise: Triceps brachii

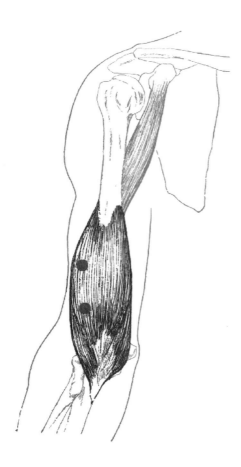

Brachialis and trigger points

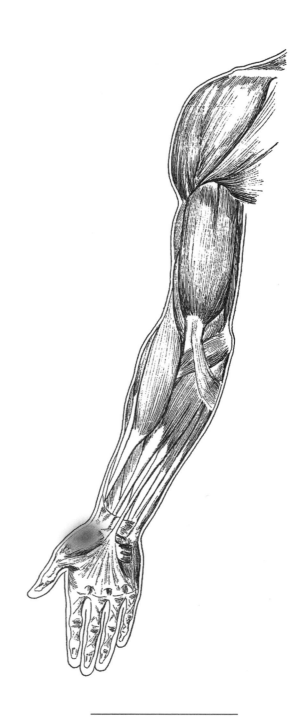

Brachialis pain pattern

BRACHIALIS

Proximal attachment: Distal one-half of the shaft of the anterior humerus.

Distal attachment: Coronoid process of the ulna.

Action: Flexion of the forearm at the elbow.

Palpation: Because of its placement on the anterior aspects of the humerus and ulna, the brachialis is the primary flexor of the forearm.

To locate brachialis, identify the following structure:

- Biceps brachii—See muscle description on page 111.

To palpate brachialis, supinate the patient's arm. Flex the arm approximately 30 degrees and move the bulk of biceps brachii medially, using the pads of the fingers. Press deep to the displaced biceps to palpate brachialis on the distal one-third of the humerus.

Pain pattern: Pain and tenderness at the base of the thumb.

Causative or perpetuating factors: Lifting heavy objects with a bent elbow.

Satellite trigger points: Brachioradialis, biceps brachii.

Affected organ systems: Respiratory and cardiovascular systems.

Associated zones, meridians, and points: Ventral zone; Hand Tai Yin Lung meridian, Hand Jue Yin Pericardium meridian, Hand Shao Yin Heart meridian; LU 5, PC 3, HE 3.

Stretch exercise: Hyperextend the supinated arm, fully extending the hand and fingers to increase the stretch of the forearm. Placement of the hand beside the seated body, with the palm down and fingers pointing back, will markedly increase the stretch. Hold this position for a count of ten to fifteen.

Strengthening exercise: Stand with the arms at the sides, palms facing outward. Flex the forearms and, keeping the elbows close to the body, draw the palms toward the shoulder. Slowly return to the starting position. Flex to a count of two; release to a count of four.

Repeat eight to ten times, increasing repetitions as strength allows. Hand weights may be used to increase the work effort placed on the muscle.

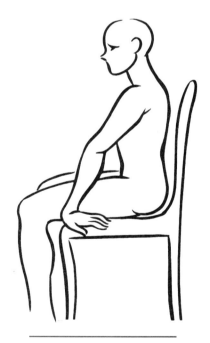

Stretch exercise: Brachialis

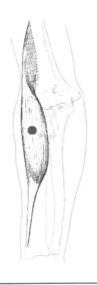

Brachioradialis and trigger point

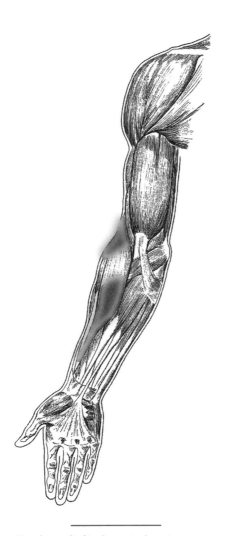

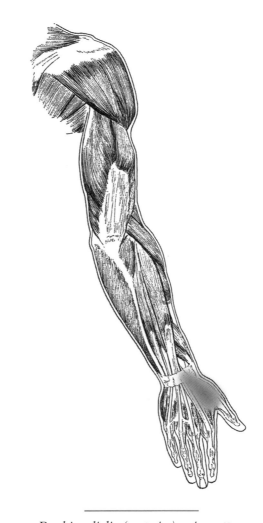

Brachioradialis (anterior) pain pattern   *Brachioradialis (posterior) pain pattern*

BRACHIORADIALIS

Proximal attachment: Lateral supracondylar ridge of the humerus and the lateral intermuscular septum at the level of the mid-arm.

Distal attachment: Styloid process of the radius.

Action: Flexion of the forearm at the elbow, expecially when the arm is in the neutral position; assists resisted pronation and supination of the forearm.

Palpation: Brachioradialis is the most superficial muscle of the lateral aspect of the forearm. It gives the upper forearm its characteristic shape.

To locate brachioradialis, identify the following structures:

- Lateral supracondylar ridge of the humerus—The vertical ridge on the lateral aspect of the humerus starting just above the lateral epicondyle
- Styloid process of the radius—The lateral, distal end of the radius

To locate brachioradialis, flex the elbow against resistance with the forearm in the neutral (midprone) position—hold a light fist and press up against the bottom of a tabletop using the index finger/thumb part of the fist. The brachioradialis becomes clearly prominent. With the forearm in the neutral position, palpate brachioradialis from its attachment on the humerus, through the muscle belly, to its tendinous attachment on the styloid process of the radius.

Pain pattern: Pain experienced at the lateral epicondyle through the length of the muscle to the web of the thumb on the dorsal aspect of the hand. The pain is often described as "tennis elbow" and is accompanied by a weak or unreliable grip.

Causative or perpetuating factors: Forceful or repetitive gripping of a large or wide object.

Satellite trigger points: Hand extensors.

Affected organ system: Respiratory system.

Associated zones, meridians, and points: Ventral zone; Hand Tai Yin Lung meridian; LU 4, 5, and 6.

Stretch exercise: With the elbow straight and the arm supinated, fully extend the wrist and place the hand in ulnar deviation.

Strengthening exercise: Stand with the arms at your sides, palms facing outward. Flex the forearms and, keeping the elbows close to the body, draw the palms toward the shoulder. Slowly return to the starting position. Flex to a count of two; release to a count of four.

Repeat eight to ten times, increasing repetitions as strength allows. Hand weights may be used to increase the work effort placed on the muscle.

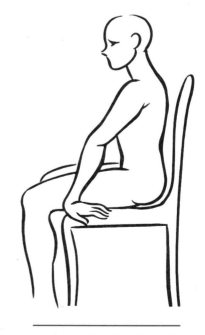

Stretch exercise: Brachioradialis

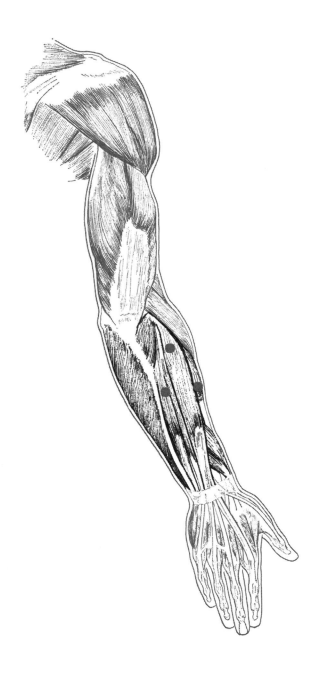

Hand and finger extensors and trigger points

Hand and Finger Extensors

Extensor carpi radialis longus, Extensor carpi radialis brevis, Extensor digitorum, Extensor digiti minimi, Extensor carpi ulnaris★

Proximal attachment: *Extensor carpi radialis longus:* lateral epicondyle of the humerus via the common extensor tendon and the lateral supracondylar ridge. *Extensor carpi radialis brevis:* lateral epicondyle of the humerus via the common extensor tendon. *Extensor digitorum:* lateral epicondyle of the humerus, intermuscular septum, and antebrachial fascia. *Extensor digiti minimi:* lateral epicondyle of the humerus via the common extensor tendon. *Extensor carpi ulnaris:* lateral epicondyle of the humerus via the common extensor tendon, and the proximal ulna.

Distal attachment: *Extensor carpi radialis longus:* base of the second metacarpal. *Extensor carpi radialis brevis:* base of the third metacarpal. *Extensor digitorum:* middle and distal phalanges of each of the four fingers. *Extensor digiti minimi:* middle and distal phalanges of the little finger. *Extensor carpi ulnaris:* base of the fifth metacarpal.

Action: *Extensor carpi radialis longus:* extension and radial deviation of the hand. *Extensor carpi radialis brevis:* extension of the hand. *Extensor digitorum:* extension of the four fingers. *Extensor digiti minimi:* extension and abduction of the little finger. *Extensor carpi ulnaris:* extension and ulnar deviation of the hand.

Palpation: Each of these superficial muscles of the dorsal forearm can harbor constrictions that may be the source of myofascial pain. It is recommended that areas of constriction be located using digital palpation along the dorsal (posterior) forearm, following the course of each muscle as it moves from its proximal position at the lateral epicondyle to the wrist and hand. In order to identify each muscle, move the hand and fingers through the actions performed by each individual muscle as you palpate.

Pain pattern: Pain over the lateral epicondyle and the dorsum of the forearm and hand and possibly throughout the fingers. Pain may be described as "tennis elbow" and may be accompanied by a weak or unreliable grip. Weakness is pronounced when the hand is in ulnar deviation.

Causative or perpetuating factors: Repetitive or forceful handgrip; "writer's cramp."

★Moving lateral to medial on the dorsal (posterior) surface of the forearm

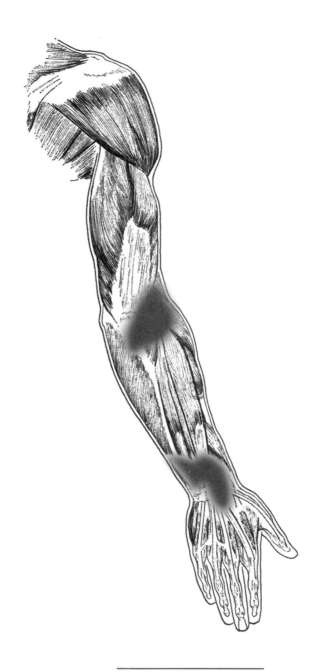

Hand and finger extensors pain pattern

Satellite trigger points: Brachioradialis.

Affected organ system: Digestive system.

Associated zones, meridians, and points: Dorsal zone; Hand Tai Yang Small Intestine meridian, Hand Yang Ming Colon meridian, Hand Shao Yang Triple Warmer meridian; SI 6, 7, and 8; CO 5–11; SJ 4–10.

Stretch exercise: Flex the wrist with the elbow fully extended. While maintaining the extended elbow, place the dorsum of the hand on a table to increase the stretch, or stabilize the flexed hand using the opposite hand.

Strengthening exercise: Form a light fist while maintaining a neutral or slightly flexed wrist position. Keeping the elbow fully extended, extend the wrist. Return to a neutral position. Repeat eight to ten times. Light hand weights may be used to increase the work effort of the hand extensors.

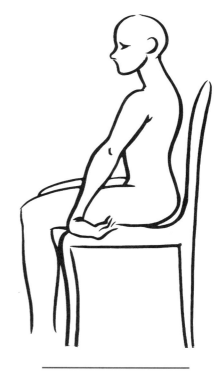

Stretch exercise: Hand extensors

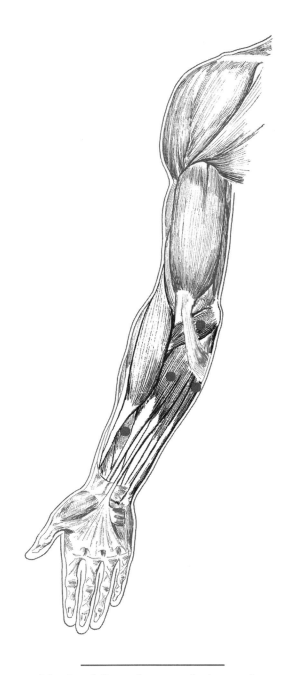

Hand and finger flexors and trigger points

HAND AND FINGER FLEXORS

FLEXOR CARPI RADIALIS, PALMARIS LONGUS, FLEXOR DIGITORUM SUPERFICIALIS, FLEXOR CARPI ULNARIS★

Proximal attachment: *Flexor carpi radialis:* medial epicondyle of the humerus via the common flexor tendon. *Palmaris longus:* medial epicondyle of the humerus via the common flexor tendon. *Flexor digitorum superficialis:* medial epicondyle of the humerus via the common flexor tendon, medial aspect of the coronoid process of the ulna, and proximal one-half of the radius. *Flexor carpi ulnaris:* medial epicondyle of the humerus via the common flexor tendon and proximal two-thirds of the posterior ulna.

Distal attachment: *Flexor carpi radialis:* base of the second and possibly the third metacarpal. *Palmaris longus:* palmar aponeurosis. *Flexor digitorum superficialis:* middle phalange of each of the four fingers. *Flexor carpi ulnaris:* pisiform bone.

Action: *Flexor carpi radialis:* flexion and radial deviation of the hand. *Palmaris longus:* flexion of the hand. *Flexor digitorum superficialis:* flexion of the middle phalange of each of the four fingers. *Flexor carpi ulnaris:* flexion and ulnar deviation of the hand.

Palpation: Each of the superficial muscles of the ventral forearm can harbor constrictions that may be the source of myofascial pain. Palpate these muscles with the forearm fully supinated and the hand and fingers extended. Locate areas of constriction using digital palpation along the ventral (anterior) forearm, following the course of each muscle as it moves from its proximal position on the forearm to the wrist and hand. In order to identify each muscle, move the hand and fingers through the actions performed by each individual muscle as you palpate. While flexor carpi radialis, palmaris longus, and flexor carpi ulnaris may be palpated throughout their course, flexor digitorum superficialis may be palpated in the distal one-third of the forearm, in between the tendons of brachioradialis and flexor carpi radialis on the radial side and between the tendons of palmaris longus and flexor carpi ulnaris on the ulnar side.

★Moving lateral to medial on the ventral (anterior) surface of the forearm.

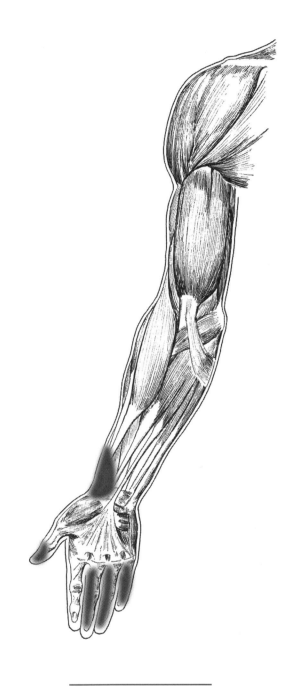

Hand and finger flexors pain pattern

Pain. pattern: Finger pain; possibly a "trigger finger," in which the interphalangeal joint locks in flexion; pain with repetitive forceful or extensive flexion of the hand and fingers; *Palmaris longus:* pain radiating into the center of the palm of the hand.

Causative or perpetuating factors: Repetitive or prolonged gripping, twisting, or pulling movements of the hand and fingers.

Satellite trigger points: Each of the hand and finger flexors may develop satellite trigger points in response to the presence of trigger points in any other muscle of the group.

Affected organ systems: Respiratory and cardiovascular systems.

Associated zones, meridians, and points: Ventral zone; Hand Tai Yin Lung meridian, Hand Jue Yin Pericardium meridian, Hand Shao Yin Heart meridian; LU 5–9, HE 3–7, PC 3–7.

Stretch exercise: Slowly press the fingers and wrist into extension using the opposite hand or by pressing the palm and fingers down onto a flat surface while keeping the elbow straight. Hold for a count of five to ten.

Strengthening exercise: Form a light fist while maintaining a neutral or slightly extended wrist position. With the elbow fully extended, flex the wrist. Return to a neutral position.

Repeat eight to ten times. Light hand weights may be used to increase the work effort of the hand flexors.

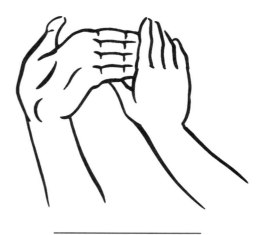

Stretch exercise: Hand and finger flexors

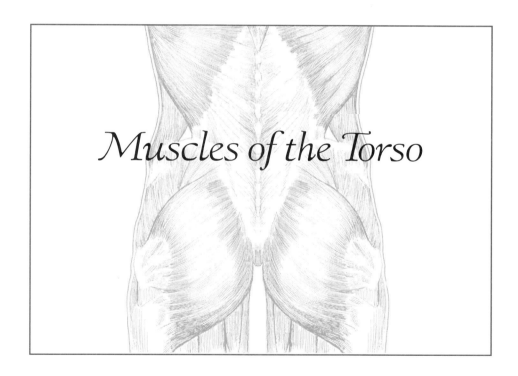

Muscles of the Torso

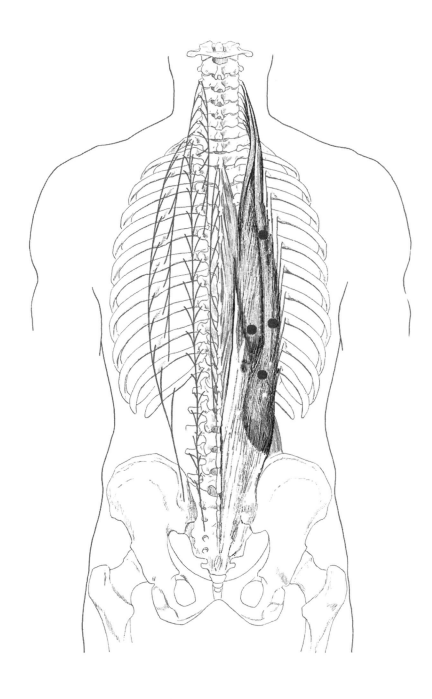

Erector spinae and trigger points

ERECTOR SPINAE

ILIOCOSTALIS THORACIS, ILIOCOSTALIS LUMBORUM, LONGISSIMUS THORACIS, SPINALIS

Of the three muscles identified as part the erector spinae group (iliocostalis, longissimus, and spinalis), iliocostalis and longissimus are considered to be the most clinically significant in most cases. The spinalis is the most medially placed muscle of the group. It is generally poorly developed and has little clinical significance; it is therefore not included in our discussion.

Proximal attachment: *Iliocostalis thoracis:* angles of the upper six ribs. *Iliocostalis lumborum:* angles of the lowest six ribs. *Longissimus thoracis:* transverse processes of all thoracic vertebrae and adjacent ribs.

Distal attachment: *Iliocostalis thoracis:* angles of the lowest six or seven ribs. *Iliocostalis lumborum* and *longissimus thoracis:* via the shared lumbocostal aponeurosis of the erector spinae, attaching to the transverse processes of the lumbar vertebrae (L1–L5) and to the sacrum, iliac crest, and spinous processes of the lumbar vertebrae.

Action: *Acting bilaterally:* extension of the trunk. *Acting unilaterally:* lateral bending to the same side. The erector spinae muscles contract strongly while coughing or straining to have a bowel movement.

Palpation: The erector spinae are the superficial layer of the paraspinal muscles. They are considered the "true" back muscles due to their work of maintaining posture and their direct action on movement of the vertebral column.

For the purpose of palpation, iliocostalis and longissimus should be considered as one group. To locate iliocostalis and longissimus, identify the following structures:

- Spinous processes of T1–T12
- Spinous processes of L1–L5. Note the change in shape and size of the lumbar spinous processes as compared to the thoracic spinous processes.
- Sacrum
- Iliac crest—Lying on a horizontal line with the junction of L4–L5

To palpate the erector spinae, place your hands parallel to the spine, fingers together, hands flat and relaxed, with your index fingers adjacent to but not touching the spinous processes. With firm but gentle pressure, palpate through the overlying trapezius and latissimus dorsi. Your hand movement follows the vertical course of fiber direction. As you move throughout the course of the muscle you may note cord- or ropelike consistency within areas of the musculature. This is a commonly found indicator of myofascial constriction.

You may begin at either end of the spine, but palpate bilaterally and throughout the course of the musculature to assess the condition of the complete muscle group. Differentiate between the superficial musculature and the deeper erector spinae by noting the direction of the muscle fibers. Note that it may be difficult to differentiate between iliocostalis and longissimus.

Focus on the palpation of iliocostalis thoracis by assessing the condition of the most laterally placed vertical bands of muscle lying lateral to T1–T12. Focus on the palpation of iliocostalis lumborum by assessing the condition of the most laterally placed vertical bands of muscle lying lateral to T7–T12 and extending downward over the lumbar region to the sacrum and iliac crests.

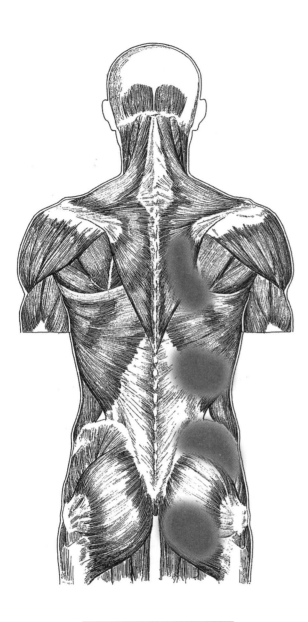

Erector spinae pain pattern

To palpate longissimus thoracis, begin close to the transverse processes of the thoracic vertebrae and the adjacent ribs. Follow fiber direction to the lumbar region where the lumbocostal aponeurosis attaches to the sacrum and iliac crests. With focused palpation, try to differentiate between the laterally placed slips of iliocostalis and the more medially placed slips of longissimus. It may be difficult to differentiate the two groups.

Pain pattern: *Iliocostalis thoracis:* pain in the thoracic region of the back and sometimes the abdomen, with restriction of spinal motion. *Iliocostalis lumborum:* pain is referred downward, low in the buttock and along the iliac crest. *Longissimus thoracis:* pain is referred low in the buttock. When trigger points are located bilaterally at the level of L1, the patient will have difficulty rising from a chair and/or climbing stairs.

Causative or perpetuating factors: Sudden overload through improper lifting; sustained overload resultant from postural stresses (hyperlordosis); immobility for extended periods of time.

Satellite trigger points: Each muscle of the erector spinae group may develop satellite trigger points in response to the presence of trigger points in any other muscle of the group. Additional trigger points might also be found in the latissimus dorsi and quadratus lumborum muscles.

Affected organ systems: Due to the placement of the *shu* (chronic disease) points along this region, constriction of regions of this muscle may reflect the condition of the following organs. *Iliocostalis thoracis:* lung, stomach, gallbladder, liver, and spleen. *Iliocostalis lumborum:* stomach, gallbladder, liver, spleen, kidney, and colon. *Longissimus thoracis:* lung, stomach, gallbladder, liver, spleen, kidney, and colon. We have observed constriction in this muscle between T6 and T12 in patients suffering with diabetes.

Associated zones, meridians, and points: Dorsal zone; Foot Tai Yang Bladder meridian; *Iliocostalis thoracis:* BL 11–21, BL 41–50; *Iliocostalis lumborum:* BL 16–26, BL 45–52; *Longissimus thoracis:* BL 11–25, BL 41–52.

Stretch exercises:

1. Seated forward stretch: Sit comfortably on a chair with the feet placed flat on the floor. Fold the torso toward the floor, reaching forward and down with the arms. Allow your head and neck to hang loosely. Hold this position for a count of twenty to thirty. Return to the seated position slowly.

2. Pelvic tilts: Lie supine. Bend the knees, placing the soles of the feet on the floor. Exhale and slowly drop the lumbar curve of the back toward the floor. Hold for a count of five, then release. Repeat several times. Be certain that the drop of the lumbar arch occurs as a result of the relaxation of the back muscles, not from an anterior tilt of the lower pelvis brought on by contracting the gluteal muscles.

3. Cats: Position the body on the hands and knees. Arch the back, lifting both the head and the buttocks toward the ceiling. Hold for a count of five. Then round the back, aiming both the head and the coccyx for the floor. Hold for a count of five. Alternate these two positions three to four times.

Strengthening exercise: Lie prone, with the hands clasped behind the head. Lift the upper portion of the body from the floor, making sure to keep the buttocks and legs relaxed. Hold for a count of one to three.

Repeat two or three times, increasing frequency and duration as the strength of the back increases.

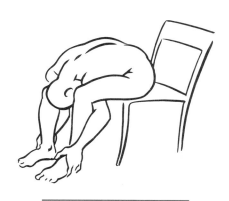

Stretch exercise 1: Erector spinae

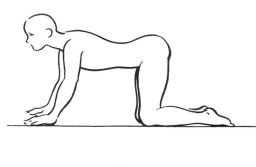

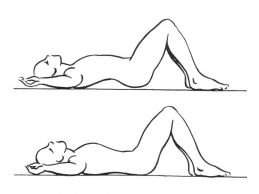

Stretch exercise 2: Erector spinae

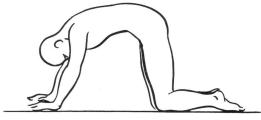

Stretch exercise 3: Erector spinae

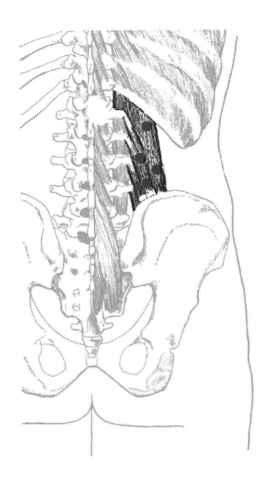

Quadratus lumborum and trigger points

QUADRATUS LUMBORUM

Proximal attachment: Medial one-half of the twelfth rib and the transverse processes of L1–L4.

Distal attachment: Uppermost posterior aspect of the crest of the ilium.

Action: *Acting unilaterally:* stabilizes the lumbar spine in the upright position; laterally flexes the lumbar spine; acts as a hip hiker. *Acting bilaterally:* extends the lumbar spine; acts in forced exhalation, as might occur in coughing; fixes the twelfth rib, facilitating contraction of the diaphragm.

Palpation: Quadratus lumborum is one of the muscles most commonly involved in lower back pain, yet it is commonly overlooked as a source.

To locate quadratus lumborum, identify the following structures:

- Rib 12—The bottommost or "floating" rib is the shortest of the twelve ribs. Locate its free anterior border posterior to the midaxillary line, level with the vertebral body of L2.
- Transverse processes of L1–L5
- Iliac crests—Lying on a horizontal line with the junction of L4–L5

Palpate quadratus lumborum with the patient lying prone. Gently depress the area between the iliac crest and the twelfth rib through the soft lateral aspect of the torso, pressing medially and obliquely toward the transverse processes of the lumbar vertebrae (not sagitally into the body). Image the location of quadratus lumborum. As you do so your hand will encounter the lateral bands of quadratus lumborum.

Pain pattern: Superficial trigger points refer pain to the lateral border of the iliac crest and over the greater trochanter. Deep trigger points refer pain over the region of the sacroiliac joint and deep within the center of the buttock. The patient may be unable to bear standing upright or walking due to deep, aching low back pain. Inability to turn over in bed without pain. Trigger points may produce an apparent leg-length discrepancy.

Causative or perpetuating factors: Overload stress of simultaneous bending and lifting; awkward lifting of heavy objects; sustained and repetitive strain; sudden leg-length discrepancy as might occur with the use of an ankle cast.

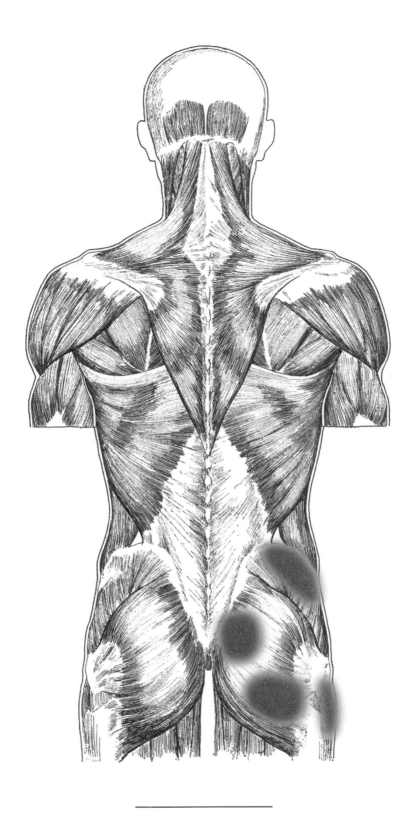

Quadratus lumborum pain pattern

Satellite trigger points: Gluteus minimus, gluteus medius, thoracolumbar paraspinals, piriformis.

Affected organ system: Kidney/genitourinary system.

Associated zones, meridians, and points: Dorsal zone; Foot Tai Yang Bladder meridian, BL 21–24, BL 51 and 52.

Stretch exercises:

1. Lying supine with the feet on the floor and the knees bent, cross the leg on the unaffected side over the leg on the affected side. Use the upper leg to gently pull the lower leg toward the floor. Hold for a count of fifteen to twenty.

2. Stand with the back approximately 12 inches away from a wall. Twist the upper body to place both palms on the wall. Hold for a count of fifteen to twenty.

3. Cross the affected leg behind the unaffected leg, shifting your weight toward the affected hip. Reach both arms above the head, grasping the wrist of the homolateral arm with the opposite hand. Laterally bend the torso toward the unaffected side. Hold this position for a count of ten to fifteen.

Strengthening exercise: Because quadratus lumborum is a postural muscle, strengthening exercises are generally not necessary.

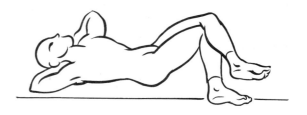

Stretch exercise 1: Quadratus lumborum

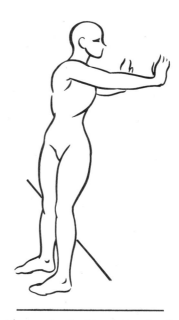

Stretch exercise 2: Quadratus lumborum

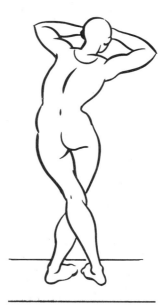

Stretch exercise 3: Quadratus lumborum

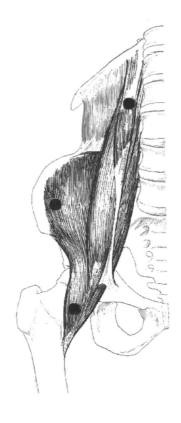

Iliopsoas and trigger points

ILIOPSOAS

Proximal attachment: Anterior bodies and intervertebral discs of T12–L5; upper two-thirds of the iliac fossa.

Distal attachment: Lesser trochanter of the femur.

Action: Flexion of the thigh at the hip when the torso is fixed; flexion of the hip on the thigh when the thigh is fixed; assists in extension of the lumbar spine (increasing lordosis) in the standing position.

Palpation: Iliopsoas is comprised of three muscles: iliacus, psoas major, and psoas minor. These are muscles of the posterior abdominal wall. Together they act as the strongest flexor of the thigh at the hip. The depth at which iliopsoas lies makes it extremely difficult to palpate these muscles throughout their course, however a small portion of the attachment onto the lesser trochanter may be palpable.

To locate iliopsoas, identify the following structures:

• Anterior superior iliac spine (ASIS)—Anterior bony projection lying somewhat below the iliac crest, readily palpable. The ASIS serves as the proximal attachment of the inguinal ligament.

• Rectus abdominis—See muscle description on page 143.

• Femoral triangle—Bounded superiorly by the inguinal ligament, medially by adductor longus (see muscle description on page 181), and laterally by sartorius (see muscle description on page 191). The floor of the femoral triangle is formed medially by pectinius and laterally by iliopsoas. Within this triangle the femoral pulse can be palpated 2 to 3 centimeters (approximately 1 inch) inferior to the inguinal ligament, at the midline of the base of the triangle that it

forms. Both the femoral artery and femoral lymph glands lie superficial to iliopsoas and pectinius, which themselves lie superficial to the hip joint. The femoral artery lies just superficial to the head of the femur. The pulse point of the femoral artery can be palpated just superficial to the head of the femur, inferior to the midpoint of the inguinal ligament.

Image the placement of iliopsoas deep within the abdomen, lying just lateral to the vertebral bodies of T12–L5, passing to the inner aspects of the ilium, and attaching to the lesser trochanter of the femur. To palpate the most distal fibers of iliopsoas, abduct the thigh, flexing the lower leg. Locate the femoral triangle. Palpate iliopsoas at the lateral aspect of the floor of the triangle, medial to sartorius and slightly distal to the inguinal ligament.

Due to the sagittal depth of this muscle, success in palpating and treating a constricted iliopsoas is somewhat elusive. However, we have found that marked changes of the iliopsoas can be obtained by affecting the iliopsoas fascia at the lateral one-half of the inguinal ligament. By using acupuncture needling or direct digital pressure close to the distal portion of the attachments of these muscles at the ASIS and the lateral aspect of the inguinal ligament, the homolateral iliopsoas can be significantly released.

Releases of constriction in the upper fibers of iliopsoas can be obtained through the application of pressure or needling techniques through the abdomen, at the level of the navel, lateral to the border of rectus abdominis. Pressure should be applied medially and obliquely toward the midline.

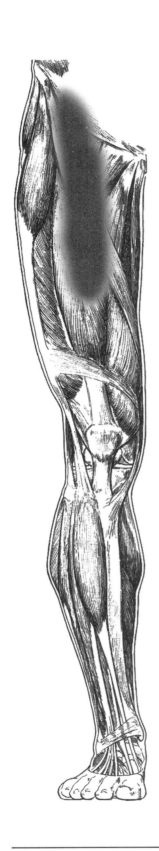

Iliopsoas (anterior) pain pattern

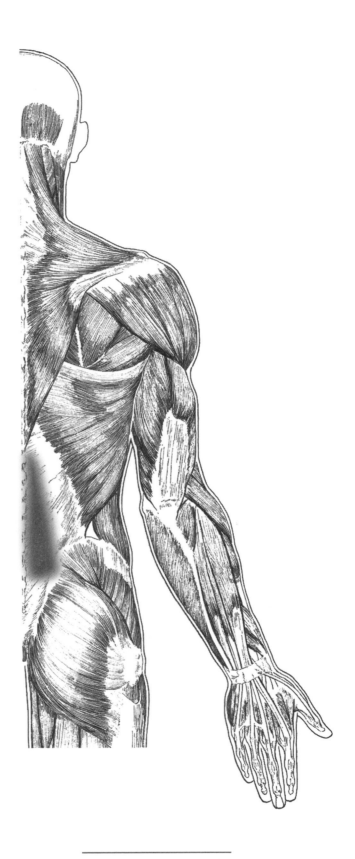

Iliopsoas (posterior) pain pattern

Pain pattern: Vertical pain that is worsened by weight-bearing activities and relieved by rest; relief is greatest when the hip is flexed. Upper trigger point refers unilaterally on the side of the trigger point with pain, extending from T12 to the ilium and upper buttock; lower trigger points refer pain to the groin and the anterior aspect of the upper thigh. Symptoms may include the inability to stand upright.

Causative or perpetuating factors: Sitting for extended periods of time with the hips acutely flexed.

Satellite trigger points: Quadratus lumborum, rectus abdominis, tensor fascia latae, gluteus maximus, gluteus medius, gluteus minimus, thoracolumbar paraspinals, piriformis.

Affected organ systems: Genitourinary and digestive systems.

Associated zones, meridians, and points: Ventral zone; Foot Yang Ming Stomach meridian, Foot Shao Yang Gall Bladder meridian; ST 25, GB 27 and 28.

Stretch exercises:

1. Lying on a table or bed, abduct the thigh and leg of the affected side and allow the limb to hang off the side of the table or bed. Flex the thigh and leg of the unaffected side to fix the pelvis, keeping the lumbar spine flat on the table or bed. Allow gravity to stretch the upper groin area. Hold for a count of twenty to thirty.

2. Cobra: Lying prone, place the hands palms down at the level of the chest. Raise the upper body, supporting it with the weight on the arms. Arch the head and neck toward the ceiling, keeping the hips, legs, and feet relaxed on the floor. Hold for a count of twenty to thirty.

   Release the stretch by relaxing the arms, bending the elbows to support the upper body weight, and slowly bringing the body down to the prone position.

Strengthening exercise: Leg lifts: Lie on the floor in the supine position. Place the hands, palms down, under the buttocks, reducing the lumbar arch and bringing it into contact with the floor. (It is essential to make certain that the lumbar region remains in contact with the floor in order to reduce the risk of injury to the back in this exercise.) From this position, raise the legs, knees slightly bent, approximately 12 inches and then return them to the starting position.

Repeat eight to ten times.

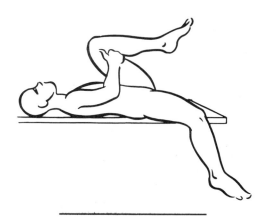

Stretch exercise 1: Iliopsoas

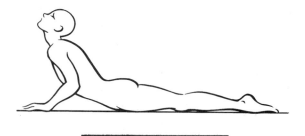

Stretch exercise 2: Iliopsoas

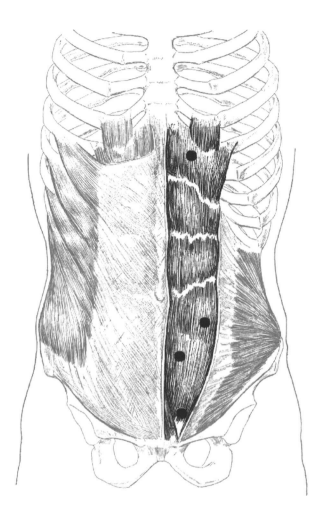

Rectus abdominis and trigger points

RECTUS ABDOMINIS

Proximal attachment: Cartilages of ribs 5, 6, and 7; xiphoid process.

Distal attachment: Crest of the pubic bone.

Action: Flexion of the trunk; upward rotation of the pelvis.

Palpation: The abdominal muscles form a continuous sheath within which lie the abdominal viscera. This sheath is bounded superiorly by the diaphragm; posteriorly by the psoas; posterolaterally by quadratus lumborum; anterolaterally by transversus abdominis, internal oblique, and external oblique (moving deep to superficial); and anteriorly by rectus abdominis. The muscles of the pelvic floor form the inferior boundary of this sheath.

By and large, rectus abdominis and the other abdominal muscles—external oblique, internal oblique, and transversus abdominis—are difficult to distinguish from one another unless one is in a state of contraction or harbors taut bands. For the purposes of the treatment of myofascial constrictions within this group it is recommended that the patient's experience of pain be the guide that directs the practitioner's hands to the areas that may harbor constrictions. That is, palpation should begin where the patient describes his pain or discomfort to be. Palpation should be gentle enough to examine the abdominal musculature without forcing through it to the underlying viscera.

To locate rectus abdominis, identify the following structures:

- Xiphoid process
- Cartilages of ribs 5, 6, and 7
- Crest of the pubic bone
- Linea alba (white line)—Tendinous union of the bilateral aponeuroses of the external oblique, internal oblique, and transversus abdominis muscles, lying deep to the skin in the midline of the torso

Palpate rectus abdominis from the proximal attachment at the costal cartilages to the distal attachment at the pubic bone, following the vertical course of the muscle fibers. Place the hands, flat and relaxed, on the abdomen, with the fingers lying parallel to the direction of rectus abdominis; note the linea alba in the midline. The lateral boundary of the rectus abdominis is readily palpable in muscularly developed people. Note the segments into which the rectus abdominis is divided. Palpate rectus abdominis throughout its course for taut bands.

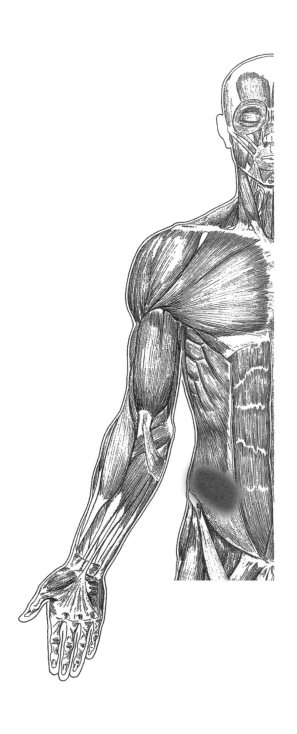

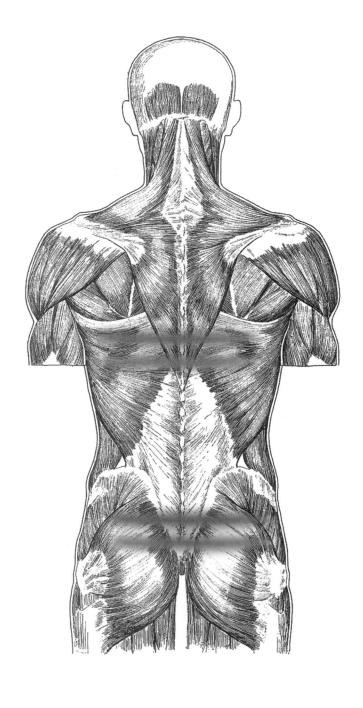

Rectus abdominis (anterior) pain pattern

Rectus abdominis (posterior) pain pattern

Pain pattern: Trigger points within the proximal aspect of the muscle may produce bilateral midback pain; trigger points within the distal aspect may produce horizontal low back pain as well as unilateral pain in the lower abdomen. Symptoms include heartburn, the sensation of abdominal fullness, indigestion, vomiting, and nausea; periumbilical involvement produces abdominal cramping. Lower trigger point involvement may result in dysmenorrhea.

Causative or perpetuating factors: Acute or chronic overload strain; muscular overuse; visceral disease; abdominal surgical scars; paradoxical breathing; poor posture.

Satellite trigger points: External oblique, internal oblique, transversus abdominis, iliocostalis thoracis, iliocostalis lumborum, longissimus thoracis, iliopsoas.

Affected organ systems: Digestive and genitourinary systems.

Associated zones, meridians, and points: Ventral zone; Foot Yang Ming Stomach meridian, Foot Shao Yin Kidney meridian; ST 19–30, KI 11–21.

Stretch exercise: Cobra: Lying prone, place the hands palms down at the level of the chest. Raise the upper body, supporting it with the weight on the arms. Arch the head and neck toward the ceiling, keeping the hips, legs, and feet relaxed on the floor. Hold for a count of fifteen to twenty. Release the stretch by relaxing the arms, bending the elbows to support the upper body weight and slowly bringing the body down to the prone position.

Strengthening exercises:

1. Roll downs: Begin in the seated position with the legs extended in front of you. Bend the knees, placing the soles of the feet on the floor. Inhale. Exhale, dropping the chin to the chest, rounding the lumbar spine, and slowly rolling backward toward the floor. First the lumbar spine touches the floor, then the thoracic spine, then the upper back, then the head. If need be you can control the backward movement of your weight by holding on to your legs as you roll back. Greater stress will be placed on the abdominal muscles the more slowly you roll down. Reverse the exercise to roll up.

2. Abdominal crunches: Lying in the supine position bend the knees, placing the soles of the feet on the floor. Clasp the hands behind the head or cross the arms on the chest. Inhale deeply. Exhale, focusing on touching the navel to the spine, and roll up by bringing the chin to chest, raising the upper body, and lifting the scapulae off the floor. Slowly roll down to the starting position. Repeat three to five times, increasing repetitions as strength allows.

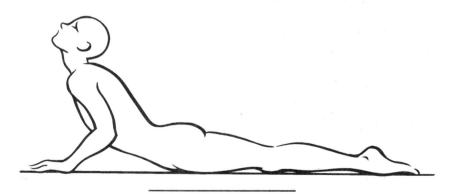

Stretch exercise: Rectus abdominis

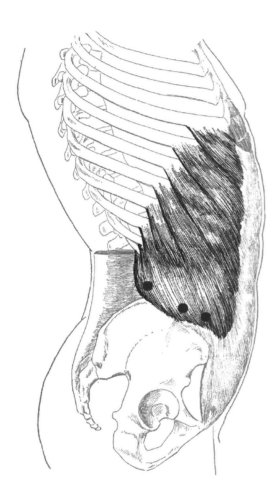

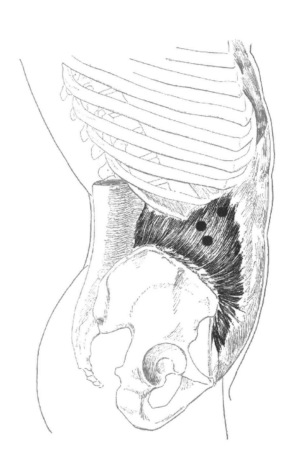

Abdominals (external oblique)
and trigger points

Abdominals (internal oblique)
and trigger points

ABDOMINALS

EXTERNAL OBLIQUE, INTERNAL OBLIQUE, TRANSVERSUS ABDOMINIS

Proximal attachment: *External oblique:* six lower ribs. *Internal oblique:* iliopsoas fascia adjacent to the lateral one-half of the inguinal ligament, anterior iliac crest, spinous and transverse processes of the five lumbar vertebrae via the thoracolumbar fascia, cartilages of ribs 9–12. *Transversus abdominis:* lumbar vertebrae via the thoracolumbar aponeurosis, the lower six ribs, anterior iliac crest, iliopsoas fascia adjacent to the lateral aspect of the inguinal ligament.

Distal attachment: *External oblique:* linea alba via an abdominal aponeurosis forming the anterior rectus sheath (passing superficial to rectus abdominis), anterior iliac crest, pubis. *Internal oblique:* linea alba via the abdominal aponeurosis forming the anterior rectus sheath (passing superficial to rectus abdominis). *Transversus abdominis:* linea alba via the abdominal aponeurosis forming the posterior rectus sheath (passing deep to rectus abdominis), pubis.

Action: Compression of the abdomen. *External oblique:* rotation of the trunk to the opposite side. Lateral flexion of the trunk to the same side when acting with the homolateral internal oblique. *Internal oblique:* lateral flexion and rotation of the trunk to the same side when acting with the contralateral external oblique.

Palpation: For general instruction on palpating the abdominal muscles, see page 143.

To locate external oblique, internal oblique, and transversus abdominis, identify the following structures:

- Ribs 7–12
- Anterior aspect of the iliac crest
- Pubic bone
- Linea alba (white line)—Tendinous union of the bilateral aponeuroses of the external

oblique, internal oblique, and transversus abdominis, lying deep to the skin in the midline of the torso

Palpate external oblique on the lateral aspect of the torso. Note that its fibers run obliquely down and medially. Begin palpation on the lateral aspect of the lower rib cage, placing your hands along the fiber direction of the muscle. Hand movement will move downward and medial to the iliac crest and toward the pubic bone. Palpation must be gentle enough to examine the musculature without forcing through it to the underlying viscera.

It may be difficult to distinguish external oblique from the underlying internal oblique and transversus abdominis; however, the right external oblique can be palpated when rotation to the left is resisted and vice versa. Ask the patient to rotate his right shoulder toward his left hip. Resist this motion at the shoulder while placing the palpating hand proximal to the iliac crest. External oblique can be palpated as it contracts to perform this movement.

Palpate internal oblique through the overlying external oblique on the lateral aspect of the torso. Note that its fibers run obliquely upward and lateral. Begin palpation on the lateral aspect of the lower rib cage, palpating toward the iliac crest and the inguinal ligament. It may be difficult to distinguish internal oblique from the overlying external oblique; however, the left internal oblique can be palpated when rotation to the left is resisted and vice versa. Ask the patient to rotate his right shoulder toward his left hip. Resist this motion at the shoulder while placing the palpating hand proximal to the iliac

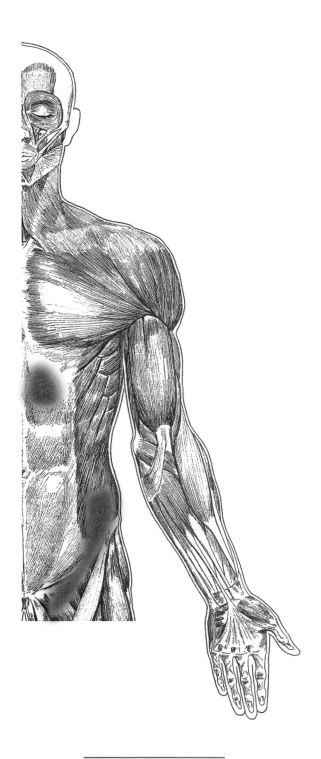

Abdominals pain pattern

crest. Internal oblique can be palpated as it contracts to perform this movement.

Transversus abdominis is obscured to palpation due to its placement deep to external oblique and internal oblique.

Pain pattern: *External oblique:* Heartburn, epigastric pain, flank pain, groin and testicular pain when trigger points are present in both transversus abdominis and internal oblique. Visceral dysfunction represents considerable symptomology associated with trigger points in the internal oblique and transversus abdominis, making pictorial representation of pain patterns unnecessary. *Internal oblique:* Symptoms are irritability and spasm of the urinary sphincter, leading to urinary frequency, retention of urine, and groin pain. *Transversus abdominis:* Symptoms are groin and testicular pain when trigger points are present in external oblique and internal oblique.

Causative or perpetuating factors: Acute or chronic overload strain; muscular overuse; abdominal surgical scars; visceral disease; paradoxical breathing; poor posture; sustained or vigorous twisting of the torso.

Satellite trigger points: Each abdominal muscle may develop satellite trigger points in response to the presence of trigger points in other muscles of the group. Additional trigger points might also be found in the iliopsoas, iliocostalis thoracis, and longissimus thoracis.

Affected organ systems: Digestive, genito-urinary, and reproductive systems.

Associated zones, meridians, and points: Ventral and lateral zones; Foot Yang Ming Stomach meridian, Foot Shao Yang Gall Bladder meridian, Foot Jue Yin Liver meridian, Foot Tai Yin Spleen meridian; SP 14, 15, and 16; LIV 13; GB 25–28.

Stretch exercises:

1. Cobra: Lying prone, place the hands palms down at the level of the chest. Raise the upper body, supporting it with the weight on the arms. Arch the head and neck toward the ceiling, keeping the hips, legs, and feet relaxed on the floor. Release the stretch by relaxing the arms, bending the elbows to support the upper body weight, and slowly bringing the body down to the prone position.

2. Stand with the back approximately 12 inches away from a wall. Twist the upper body and place both palms on the wall. Hold for a count of fifteen to twenty. Note: To stretch the right external oblique the patient must turn toward the right; to stretch the right internal oblique, the patient must turn toward the left.

Strengthening exercises:

Transverse crunches: Lying in the supine position, bend the knees and place the soles of the feet on the floor. Clasp the hands behind the head or cross the arms on the chest. Inhale deeply. Exhale, focusing on touching the navel to the spine, and roll up by bringing the chin to chest, raising the upper body, and lifting the scapulae off the floor. Twist the body, aiming the right shoulder for the left hip. Slowly roll down to the starting position. Repeat the exercise, this time aiming the left shoulder for the right hip.

Repeat the set (left/right) three to five times, increasing repetitions as strength allows.

For strengthening the abdominals as a group, you can also do the following two exercises.

1. Roll downs: Begin in the seated position with the legs extended in front of you. Bend the knees, placing the soles of the feet on the floor. Inhale. Exhale, dropping the chin to the chest, rounding the lumbar spine, and slowly rolling backward toward the floor. First the lumbar spine touches the floor, then the thoracic spine, then the upper back, then the head. If need be you can control the backward movement of your weight by holding on to your legs as you roll back. Greater stress will be placed on the abdominal muscles the more slowly you roll down. Reverse the exercise to roll up.

2. Abdominal crunches: Lying in the supine position bend the knees, placing the soles of the feet on the floor. Clasp the hands behind the head or cross the arms on the chest. Inhale deeply. Exhale, focusing on touching the navel to the spine, and roll up by bringing the chin to chest, raising the upper body, and lifting the scapulae off the floor. Slowly roll down to the starting position. Repeat three to five times, increasing repetitions as strength allows.

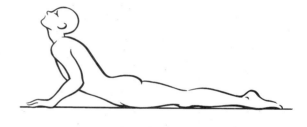

Stretch exercise 1: Abdominals

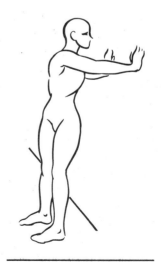

Stretch exercise 2: Abdominals

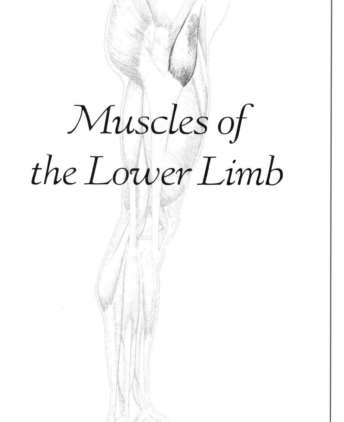

Muscles of
the Lower Limb

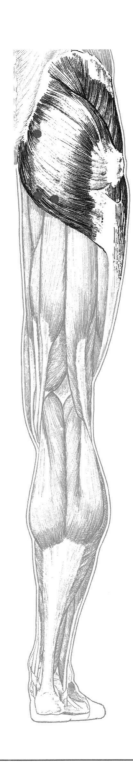

Gluteus maximus and trigger points

Gluteus Maximus

Proximal attachment: Posterior iliac crest, lateral sacrum, and coccyx.

Distal attachment: Iliotibial band of the fasciae latae and the gluteal tuberosity of the femur.

Action: Powerful extension of the thigh at the hip during strenuous activities such as running, jumping, stair climbing, and in rising from a seated position; helps maintain an erect posture; assists in lateral rotation of the hip. *Upper fibers:* abduction of the thigh. *Lower fibers:* adduction of the thigh.

Palpation: To locate gluteus maximus, identify the following structures:

- Posterior superior iliac spine (PSIS)—Bony prominence lying deep to the characteristic dimples above the buttocks. The PSIS lie horizontal to the second sacral segment. Each is approximately 2 centimeters (3/4 inch) below the superior border of the sacrum.
- Iliac crest—Lying on a horizontal line with the junction of L4–L5.

- Sacrum
- Coccyx
- Greater trochanter—Bony prominence on the lateral aspect of the femur, approximately one hand-length below the iliac crest. From the anterior plane the greater trochanter lies horizontal with the pubic crest.
- Ischial tuberosity—Easily palpable when seated, this bony prominence carries most of the weight of the torso in the seated position. It is located at the center of the buttock, approximately level with the gluteal fold.

To locate gluteus maximus, approximate its borders as follows: image its superior border by visualizing a line drawn from the PSIS to slightly above the greater trochanter; image its inferior border by visualizing a line drawn from the coccyx to the ischial tuberosity. To palpate gluteus maximus, follow the direction of muscle fibers obliquely and laterally, moving from the lateral margin of the sacrum to the greater trochanter.

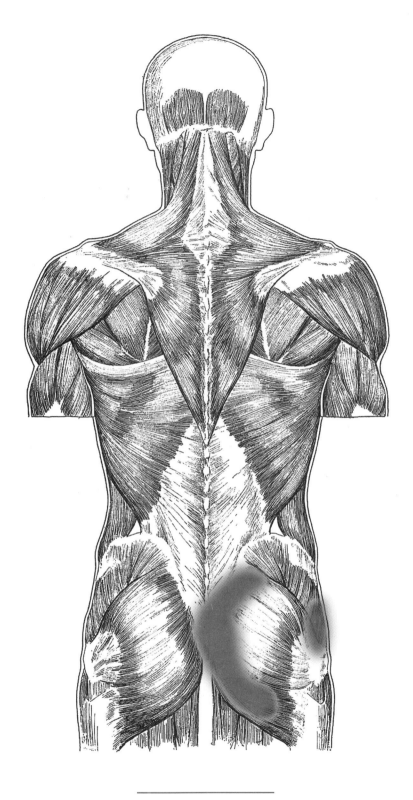

Gluteus maximus pain pattern

Pain pattern: Medial trigger points, located adjacent to the sacrum, refer pain beside the gluteal cleft, including the sacroiliac joint. Distal trigger points, located above the ischial tuberosity, refer pain throughout the buttock, including tenderness deep within the buttock. Symptoms include local pain from prolonged sitting and increased pain when walking uphill in a forward-leaning position.

Causative or perpetuating factors: Stress overload or impact from trauma or fall; prolonged walking in a forward-leaning position; injection.

Satellite trigger points: Posterior gluteus medius, posterior gluteus minimus, hamstrings, iliopsoas, rectus femoris.

Affected organ system: Elimination aspect of the digestive system; colon.

Associated zones, meridians, and points: Dorsal and lateral zones; Foot Tai Yang Bladder meridian, Foot Shao Yang Gall Bladder meridian; BL 26–30, 35 and 36, 53 and 54, GB 30.

Stretch exercise: Lying supine, draw the knee toward the homolateral shoulder, grasping the posterior thigh; pull the thigh and leg toward the shoulder, stretching the gluteus maximus. Hold for a count of ten to fifteen. Release. Then draw the knee toward the opposite shoulder. Hold for a count of ten to fifteen and release.

Strengthening exercise: Posterior pulses with a bent knee: Flex the leg of the affected side. Contract the gluteus maximus to extend the thigh. Repeat ten to twelve times.

Patient positioning will determine the degree of stress placed on the muscle. *Phase I (patient in the weakest condition):* Instruct the patient to do this exercise in the standing position, supporting his balance by holding onto a wall or chair. *Phase II:* Patient can be positioned side-lying, working the gluteal muscle of the upper leg. *Phase III:* Patient can be positioned on his hands and knees. Pulses will be working against gravity and will require the most force.

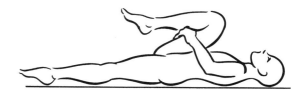

*Stretch exercise: Gluteus maximus
(knee to homolateral shoulder)*

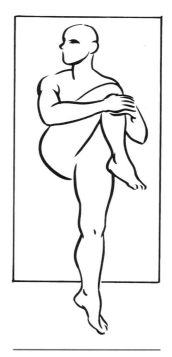

*Stretch exercise: Gluteus maximus
(knee to opposite shoulder)*

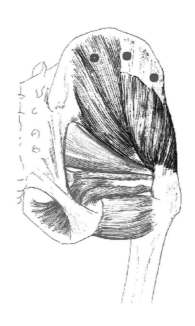

Gluteus medius and trigger points

GLUTEUS MEDIUS

Proximal attachment: Anterior three-quarters of the iliac crest.

Distal attachment: Greater trochanter of the femur.

Action: Abduction of the thigh; assists in medial rotation of the thigh. Anterior fibers flex and internally rotate the thigh; posterior fibers extend and externally rotate the thigh. Stabilizes the pelvis during ambulation.

Palpation: The posterior portion of this muscle lies deep to gluteus maximus; the anterior portion lies anterior to gluteus maximus and is superficial. Portions of this muscle lie both anterior and posterior to the hip joint. Gluteus medius is a frequently overlooked source of back pain.

To locate gluteus medius, identify the following structures:

- Iliac crest—Lying on a horizontal line with the junction of L4–L5.
- Greater trochanter—Bony prominence on the lateral aspect of the femur, approximately one hand-length below the iliac crest. From

the anterior plane the greater trochanter lies horizontal with the pubic crest.

- Anterior superior iliac spine (ASIS)— Anterior bony projection lying somewhat below the iliac crest, readily palpable. The ASIS serves as the proximal attachment for the inguinal ligament.
- Piriformis line—An imaginary line drawn from the second sacral segment (just medial to the posterior superior iliac spine [PSIS]) to the upper border of the greater trochanter. This line represents the superior border of the piriformis muscle and the posterior border of the gluteus medius muscle.

Palpate gluteus medius with the patient positioned either prone or side-lying. Palpate with flat digital pressure just distal to the iliac crest, following its course on either side of the hip joint. Areas of constriction of gluteus medius can be palpated throughout the course of the external ilium.

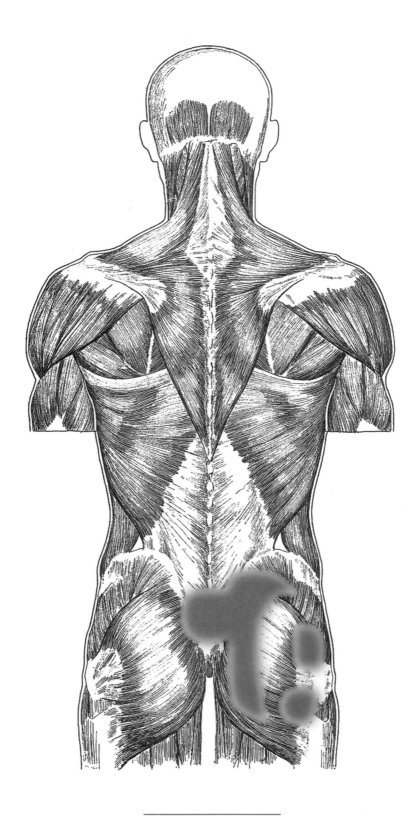

Gluteus medius pain pattern

Pain pattern: Medial trigger points refer pain to the crest of the ilium, the sacroiliac joint, and the sacrum. Lateral trigger points refer pain to the buttock and possibly the upper lateral posterior thigh. Anterior trigger points may refer bilaterally over the sacrum and the lower lumbar region. Symptoms include pain when walking, when lying on the back or on the affected side, and when sitting slouched in a chair.

Causative or perpetuating factors: Overuse injuries; sudden overload; chronic overload due to prolonged flexion of the hip; leg-length discrepancies; sacroiliac joint dysfunction.

Satellite trigger points: Quadratus lumborum, gluteus minimus, piriformis, tensor fasciae latae.

Affected organ system: Genitourinary system.

Associated zones, meridians, and points: Lateral zone; Foot Shao Yang Gall Bladder meridian; GB 29 and 30.

Stretch exercises:
1. Cross the affected leg behind the unaffected leg, shifting your weight toward the affected hip. Reach both arms above the head, grasping the wrist of the homolateral arm with the opposite hand. Laterally bend the torso toward the unaffected side. Hold this position for a count of ten to fifteen.
2. Support your balance by holding on to a wall or table. Cross the affected leg behind the unaffected leg. Bend the knee of the unaffected leg as you slide the affected leg away from the torso, toward the opposite side, aiming the hip for the floor. Hold this position for a count of ten to fifteen.

Strengthening exercise: Positioned on the hands and knees, shift your weight onto one knee, allowing freedom of motion of the working thigh and leg. Keeping the knee of the working leg bent, abduct the leg to bring the inner thigh parallel with the floor. Return the leg to the starting position. Repeat five to ten times.

Walking is one of the best exercises for this muscle.

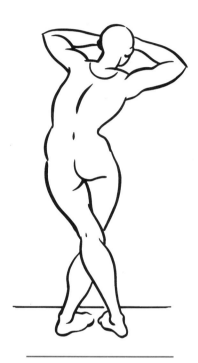

Stretch exercise 1: Gluteus medius

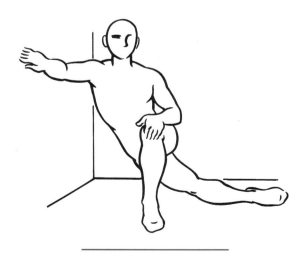

Stretch exercise 2: Gluteus medius

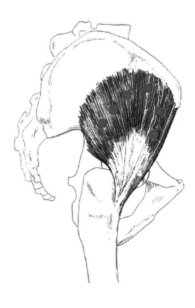

Gluteus minimus and trigger points

GLUTEUS MINIMUS

Proximal attachment: On the ilium, between the anterior and inferior gluteal lines, deep to gluteus medius.

Distal attachment: Upper aspect of the greater trochanter of the femur.

Action: Abduction of the thigh; internal rotation of the thigh. Stabilizes the pelvis during ambulation.

Palpation: Gluteus minimus, the smallest of the three gluteal muscles, lies deep to gluteus medius and tensor fasciae latae. The fiber arrangements of gluteus medius and gluteus minimus are quite similar; consequently, their actions, stretches, and strengthening exercises are very much the same.

To locate gluteus miminus, identify the following structures:

- Iliac crest—Lying on a horizontal line with the junction of L4–L5.
- Anterior superior iliac spine (ASIS)—Anterior bony projection lying somewhat below the iliac crest, readily palpable. The ASIS serves as the proximal attachment of the inguinal ligament.
- Gluteus medius—See muscle description on page 157.
- Tensor fasciae latae—See muscle description on page 165.

- Piriformis line—An imaginary line drawn from the second sacral segment (just medial to the posterior superior iliac spine [PSIS]) to the upper border of the greater trochanter. This line represents the superior border of the piriformis muscle and the lower posterior border of the gluteus medius muscle.

To locate the anterior fibers of gluteus minimus, begin with the patient lying in the supine position. Palpate just distal and lateral to the ASIS, palpating deeply both anterior to and posterior to the tensor fasciae latae. Taut bands of constricted muscle lying deep to the superficial musculature may be encountered with deep palpation.

To locate the posterior fibers of gluteus minimus, begin with the patient lying prone. Taut bands of constricted muscle may be palpated deep to the gluteus medius just superior and lateral to the midpoint of the piriformis line. Although palpating deeply, it is essential to use caution to avoid causing undue pain to the patient or injury to the superficial musculature.

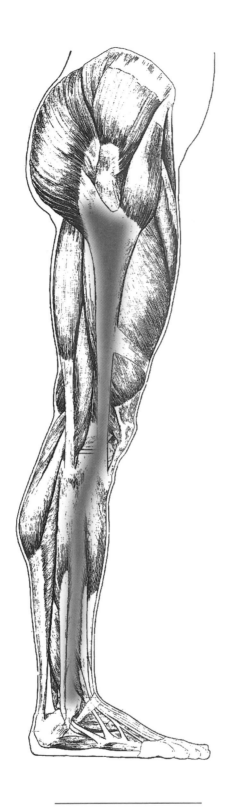

Gluteus minimus (lateral)
pain pattern

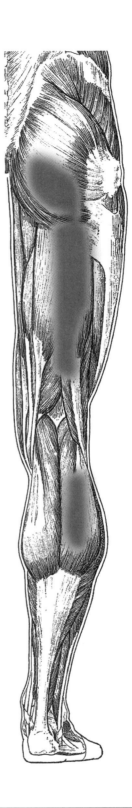

Gluteus minimus (posterior)
pain pattern

Pain pattern: Anterior trigger points refer pain to the lower lateral part of the buttock, the lateral aspect of the thigh and knee, and the lateral aspect of the leg as far as the ankle; posterior trigger points refer to the buttock, the posterior thigh and calf, and sometimes to the back of the knee. Symptoms include hip pain that may cause a limp during walking; pain while lying on the same side; pain upon rising from a chair; pain while standing straight or standing still. The pain pattern displayed by this muscle when it harbors trigger points closely resembles what is commonly referred to as sciatica.

Causative or perpetuating factors: Sudden, acute, or chronic repetitive overload; sacroiliac joint dysfunction; gait distortion; leg-length discrepancies.

Satellite trigger points: Piriformis, gluteus medius, vastus lateralis, quadratus lumborum, gluteus maximus.

Affected organ system: Genitourinary system.

Associated zones, meridians, and points: Lateral zone; Foot Shao Yang Gall Bladder meridian; GB 29 and 30.

Stretch exercises:

1. Cross the affected leg behind the unaffected leg, shifting your weight toward the affected hip. Reach both arms above the head, grasping the wrist of the homolateral arm with the opposite hand. Laterally bend the torso toward the unaffected side. Hold this position for a count of ten to fifteen.

2. Support your balance by holding onto a wall or table. Cross the affected leg behind the unaffected leg. Bend the knee of the unaffected leg as you slide the affected leg away from the torso, toward the opposite side, aiming the hip for the floor. Hold this position for a count of ten to fifteen.

Strengthening exercise: Positioned on the hands and knees, shift your weight onto one knee, allowing freedom of motion of the working thigh and leg. Keeping the knee of the working leg bent, abduct the leg to bring the inner thigh parallel with the floor. Return the leg to the starting position. Repeat five to ten times.

Walking is one of the best exercises for this muscle.

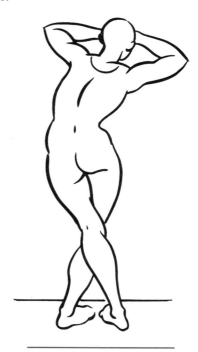

Stretch exercise 1: Gluteus minimus

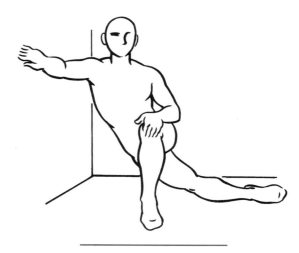

Stretch exercise 2: Gluteus minimus

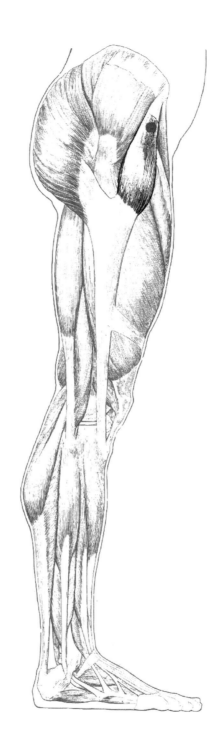

Tensor fasciae latae and trigger point

TENSOR FASCIAE LATAE

Proximal attachment: Anterior iliac crest, just posterior to the anterior superior iliac spine (ASIS).

Distal attachment: Through the iliotibial band to the lateral condyle of the tibia.

Action: Assists flexion, abduction, and internal rotation of the thigh; helps stabilize the knee. Aids gluteus medius and gluteus minimus in stabilizing the pelvis during walking.

Palpation: To locate tensor fasciae latae, identify the following structures:

- Anterior superior iliac spine (ASIS)— Anterior bony projection lying somewhat below the iliac crest, readily palpable. The ASIS serves as the proximal attachment of the inguinal ligament.
- Greater trochanter—Bony prominence on the lateral aspect of the femur, approximately one hand-length below the iliac crest. From the anterior plane the greater trochanter lies horizontal with the pubic crest.

- Iliotibial band—A long, thin, flat band of fascia lying on the outer surface of the thigh. The iliotibial band is a thickening of the normal fascia that surrounds the thigh; its distal end inserts onto the lateral condyle of the tibia. The insertion onto the lateral condyle can be palpated anterior to the insertion of the biceps femoris tendon (see muscle description on page 173). The iliotibial band can be palpated in the seated position by raising the heel of your foot off the floor while keeping your knee flexed.

To locate tensor fasciae latae place the patient in the supine position. Have him internally rotate the thigh against mild resistance; tensor fasciae latae should become readily palpable. Using flat digital palpation, follow the attachment at the ASIS to the connection with the iliotibial band on the lateral aspect of the thigh, where the fibers become tendinous. Tensor fasciae latae lies anterior to the greater trochanter of the femur.

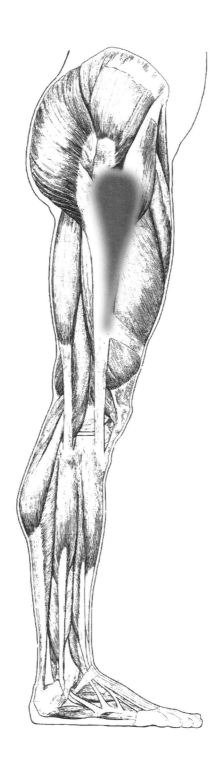

Tensor fasciae latae pain pattern

Pain pattern: Pain deep in the hip and down the lateral aspect of the thigh toward the knee. Pain may feel like the sensations associated with trochanteric bursitis. Pain prevents walking rapidly or lying comfortably on the affected side, and may interfere with the ability to sit with the hip fully flexed.

Causative or perpetuating factors: Walking or running on an uneven surface; immobilization of the limb for extended periods of time; sudden overload.

Satellite trigger points: Anterior fibers of the gluteus minimus, rectus femoris, iliopsoas, sartorius.

Affected organ system: Genitourinary system.

Associated zones, meridians, and points: Lateral zone; Foot Shao Yang Gall Bladder meridian; GB 29, GB 31.

Stretch exercises:

1. Stand or sit on the edge of a chair. Flex the lower leg, externally rotating the thigh, and grasp the ankle with the homolateral hand. Draw the heel toward the buttock, extending the thigh and hip as far as possible. Hold for a count of ten to fifteen.

2. Support your balance by holding on to a wall or table. Cross the affected leg behind the unaffected leg. Bend the knee of the unaffected leg as you slide the affected leg away from the torso, toward the opposite side, aiming the lateral hip for the floor. Hold this position for a count of ten to fifteen.

Strengthening exercise: Positioned on the hands and knees, shift your weight onto one knee, allowing freedom of motion of the working thigh and leg. Keeping the knee of the working leg bent, abduct the leg to bring the inner thigh parallel with the floor. Return the leg to the starting position. Repeat five to ten times.

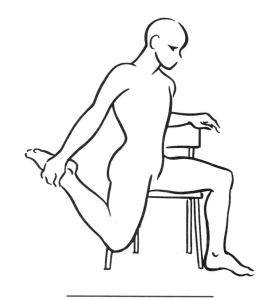

Stretch exercise 1: Tensor fasciae latae

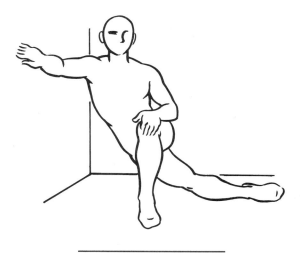

Stretch exercise 2: Tensor fasciae latae

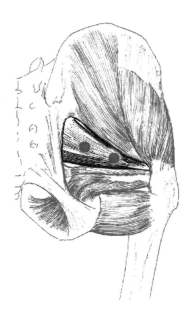

Piriformis and trigger points

PIRIFORMIS

Proximal attachment: Anterior surface of the sacrum.

Distal attachment: Through the sciatic foramen, attaching to the greater trochanter of the femur.

Action: External rotation of the thigh; acts in abduction when the thigh is flexed to 90 degrees.

Palpation: To locate piriformis, identify the following structures:

• Greater trochanter—Bony prominence on the lateral aspect of the femur, approximately one hand-length below the iliac crest. From the anterior plane the greater trochanter lies horizontal with the pubic crest.

• Piriformis line—An imaginary line drawn from the second sacral segment (just medial to the posterior superior iliac spine [PSIS]) to the upper border of the greater trochanter. This line represents the superior border of the piriformis muscle and the posterior border of the gluteus medius muscle.

Palpate piriformis with the patient side-lying or prone. Image the piriformis line; palpate slightly distal to that line, since it marks the superior border of the piriformis muscle. Palpate the muscle throughout its course, from the border of the sacrum to the greater trochanter. Taut bands of a constricted piriformis muscle can be palpated through gluteus maximus. Areas of constriction are most likely to develop in the medial aspect of the lateral one-third of the piriformis line and the lateral aspect of the medial one-third of that line.

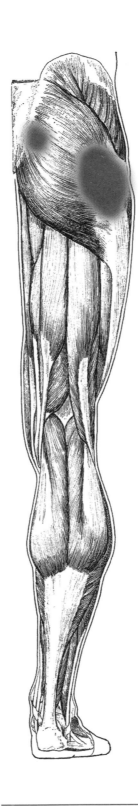

Piriformis pain pattern

Pain pattern: Pain in the sacroiliac region, the buttock, the posterior aspect of the hip joint, and possibly the proximal two-thirds of the posterior thigh. Pain is increased by sitting, standing, and walking.

Causative or perpetuating factors: Acute overload; sustained overload due to immobilization in the externally rotated position; arthritis of the hip joint; pelvic inflammatory disease.

Satellite trigger points: Gluteus medius, gluteus minimus.

Affected organ systems: Genitourinary system; elimination aspect of the digestive system.

Associated zones, meridians, and points: Dorsal and lateral zones; Foot Tai Yang Bladder meridian, Foot Shao Yang Gall Bladder meridian; GB 30.

Stretch exercise: Lying supine with the feet on the floor and the knees bent, cross the leg on the unaffected side over the leg on the affected side. Use the upper leg to gently pull the lower leg toward the floor. To ensure that the hip does not rise off the floor or table, the patient may gently apply downward pressure to the anterior superior iliac spine (ASIS) on the affected side with his hand. Hold for a count of fifteen to twenty.

Strengthening exercise: Positioned on the hands and knees, shift your weight onto one knee, allowing freedom of motion of the working thigh and leg. Keeping the knee of the working leg bent, abduct the leg to bring the inner thigh parallel with the floor. Return the leg to the starting position. Repeat five to ten times.

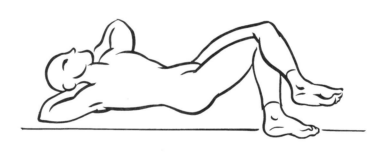

Stretch exercise: Piriformis

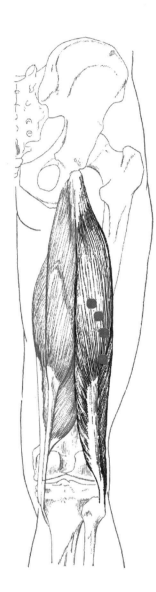 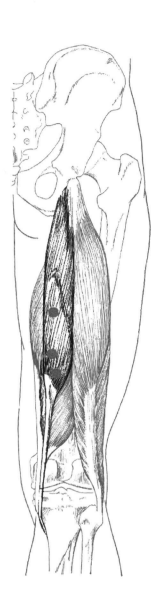 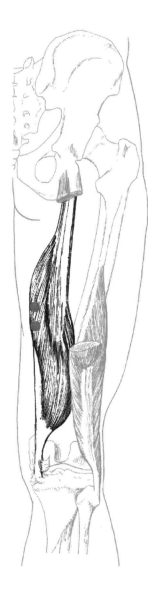

Biceps femoris   *Semitendinosus*   *Semimembranosus*

Hamstrings and trigger points

HAMSTRINGS

BICEPS FEMORIS, SEMITENDINOSUS, SEMIMEMBRANOSUS

Proximal attachment: *Biceps femoris, long head:* ischial tuberosity, by a common tendon with semitendinosus. *Biceps femoris, short head:* linea aspera of the femur, along the same portion to which the adductor magnus attaches. *Semitendinosus:* on the ischial tuberosity, by a common tendon with the long head of biceps femoris. *Semimembranosus:* on the ischial tuberosity, lateral and deep to the common tendon of biceps femoris and semitendinosus.

Distal attachment: *Biceps femoris:* both long and short heads attach by a common tendon to the posterior and lateral aspects of the head of the fibula. *Semitendinosus:* medial side of the superior part of the tibia, medial and superficial to semimembranosus, forming the pes anserinus with sartorius and gracilis. *Semimembranosus:* posterior aspect of the medial condyle of the tibia, deep to semitendinosus.

Action: *Biceps femoris, long head:* extension of the thigh. *Biceps femoris, both heads:* flexion of the leg, external rotation of the flexed leg. *Semitendinosus and semimembranosus:* extension of the thigh and flexion of the leg; assists in internal rotation of the leg at the knee.

Palpation: To locate the hamstrings, identify the following structures:

- Ischial tuberosity—Easily palpable when seated, this bony prominence carries most of the weight of the torso in the seated position. It is located at the center of the buttock, approximately level with the gluteal fold.

- Popliteal fossa—Posterior aspect of the knee joint, which appears as a hollow when the knee is flexed. It is bordered laterally by the tendon of biceps femoris and medially by the tendon of semitendinosus. As you slowly extend the leg you can palpate the fleshy semimembranosus, lying deep to semitendinosus, as it bulges posteriorly and laterally.

Palpate the hamstring group with the patient lying prone. By flexing the leg against resistance the tendons of distal attachment of both the biceps femoris, lying laterally, and the semitendinosus, lying medially, are readily observed.

Palpate biceps femoris through its course, from attachment at the ischial tuberosity to attachment on the head of the fibula. The bulk of semitendinosus fibers lie on the proximal one-half of the medial aspect of the femur, where they can be palpated along their course. Palpate semitendinosus from its attachment at the ischial tuberosity to its attachment on the proximal tibia. The bulk of semimembranosus fibers lie on the distal one-half of the medial aspect of the femur. Semimembranosus fibers can be palpated here, lying deep to semitendinosus, which is less prominent at this portion of the thigh. Semimembranosus remains muscular through to its attachment deep to semitendinosus; its tendon of insertion is not readily palpable.

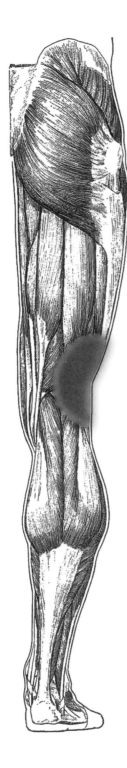

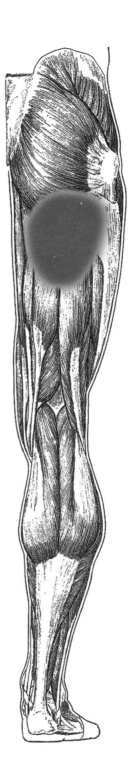

Biceps femoris

*Semitendinosus
and Semimembranosus*

Hamstrings pain pattern

Pain pattern: *Biceps femoris:* deep aching pain at the posterior and/or lateral knee, possibly extending up the posterior lateral thigh toward the gluteal fold. *Semitendinosus and semimembranosus:* pain in the lower buttock and upper thigh. Pain may extend to the posterior medial thigh and knee, as well as the proximal one-half of the medial calf.

Causative or perpetuating factors: Compression of the posterior thigh, which may occur while sitting for extended periods of time or in a poorly sized chair.

Satellite trigger points: Each muscle of the hamstring group may develop satellite trigger points in response to the presence of trigger points in any other muscle of the group. Additional satellite trigger points could also appear in adductor magnus, iliopsoas, quadriceps, quadratus lumborum, paraspinals, and rectus abdominis.

Affected organ system: Genitourinary system.

Associated zones, meridians, and points: Dorsal zone; Foot Tai Yang Bladder meridian; BL 36–40. *Semitendinosus and semimembranosus:* also Foot Shao Yin Kidney meridian; KI 10.

Stretch exercises: The short head of the biceps femoris forms a functional hamstring with adductor magnus. Therapeutic stretching of the hamstring group must therefore coincide with therapeutic stretching of the adductor group in order for each muscle group to obtain full benefit. (See page 183.)

1. Place the heel of the leg to be stretched on a step, ledge, or chair. Lean forward slowly, keeping the thigh and hips square. The higher the step, ledge, or chair the greater the stretch on this muscle group. Hold for a count of twenty to thirty, then release.
2. In standing, cross the ankles; keep the knees straight and the weight evenly distributed. Bend forward from the hips,

maintaining full extension through the knees. Hold for a count of twenty to thirty, then release.

Strengthening exercise: Lying prone, flex the working leg to a count of two; extend it to return to the prone position to a count of four. The pelvis must remain flat on the floor throughout this exercise. Repeat eight to ten times.

Ankle weights may be used to increase the demand placed on the hamstrings during this exercise. The amount of weight used must be gauged in accordance with the needs and capabilities of the patient.

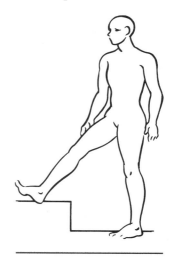

Stretch exercise 1: Hamstrings

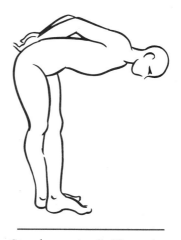

Stretch exercise 2: Hamstrings

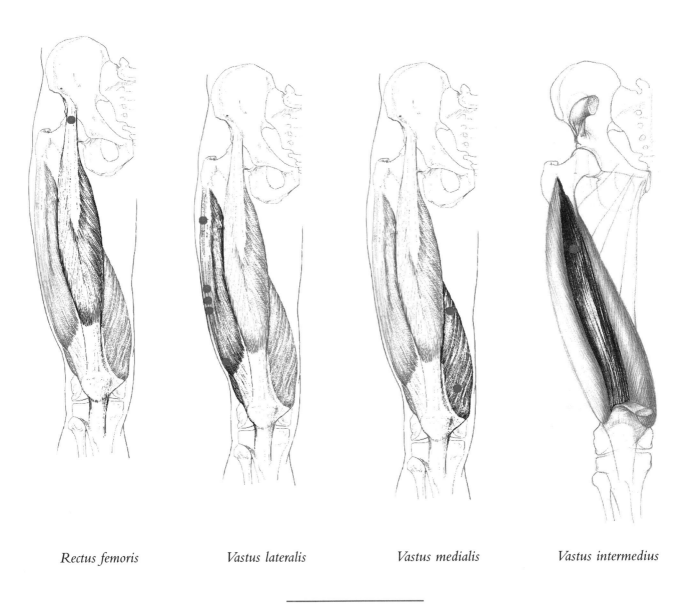

Rectus femoris   *Vastus lateralis*   *Vastus medialis*   *Vastus intermedius*

Quadriceps and trigger points

QUADRICEPS
RECTUS FEMORIS, VASTUS LATERALIS, VASTUS MEDIALIS, VASTUS INTERMEDIUS

Proximal attachment: *Rectus femoris:* via two tendons, one at the anterior superior iliac spine (ASIS) and the other at the ilium, superior to the acetabulum. *Vastus lateralis:* lateral side of the upper three-quarters of the posterior femur and the linea aspera on the posterior femur. *Vastus medialis:* full length of the posteromedial aspect of the shaft of the femur. *Vastus intermedius:* anterior and lateral surfaces of the upper two-thirds of the shaft of the femur.

Distal attachment: All quadriceps attach to the patella by means of a common tendon via the patellar ligament to the tibial tuberosity.

Action: *Rectus femoris:* extension of the leg; flexion of the thigh on the pelvis when the pelvis is fixed; flexion of the pelvis on the thigh when the thigh is fixed. *Vastus lateralis, vastus medialis, and vastus intermedius:* extension of the leg at the knee. Vastus lateralis and vastus medialis working together help to maintain normal position and tracking of the patella.

Palpation: The quadriceps group, the "great extensor," is the heaviest muscle in the body, weighing approximately 50 percent more than the next largest muscle, the gluteus maximus. Rectus femoris, vastus lateralis, and vastus medialis are readily palpable. Vastus intermedius lies deep to rectus femoris and cannot be directly palpated.

Of the four muscles that comprise the quadriceps group, only rectus femoris crosses two joints (the knee and the hip). Therefore, in addition to being an extensor of the leg, rectus femoris is a flexor of the thigh and pelvis.

To locate the quadriceps, identify the following structures:

- Anterior superior iliac spine (ASIS)— Anterior bony projection lying somewhat below the iliac crest, readily palpable. The ASIS serves as the proximal attachment of the inguinal ligament.
- Greater trochanter—Bony prominence of the lateral aspect of the femur, approximately one hand-length below the iliac crest. From the anterior plane the greater trochanter lies horizontal with the pubic crest.
- Iliotibial band—A long, thin, flat band of fascia lying on the outer surface of the thigh. The iliotibial band is a thickening of the normal fascia that surrounds the thigh; its distal end inserts onto the lateral condyle of the tibia. The insertion onto the lateral condyle can be palpated anterior to the insertion of the biceps femoris tendon (see muscle description on page 173). The iliotibial band can be palpated in the seated position by raising the heel of your foot off the floor while keeping your knee flexed.
- Patella—A sesamoid bone in the common tendon of the quadriceps group
- Tibial tuberosity

Locate rectus femoris, vastus lateralis, and vastus medialis when the leg is extended against resistance. Palpate rectus femoris from its attachment on the anterior superior iliac spine (ASIS) to its attachment via the common tendon to the tibial tuberosity.

The bulk of vastus lateralis lies proximal to the bulk of vastus medialis. Palpate the fleshy portions of vastus lateralis along the anterolateral aspect of the thigh, anterior to the iliotibial band, from the greater trochanter through its attachment via the common tendon. Palpate the fleshy portions of vastus medialis along the anteromedial aspect of the thigh through its attachment via the common tendon.

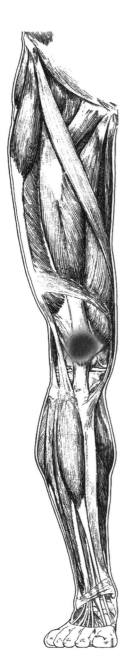

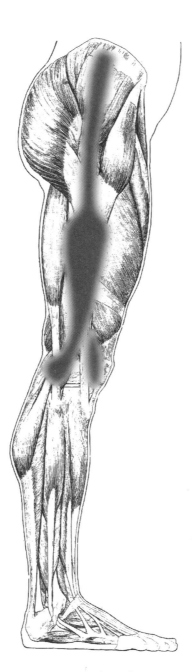

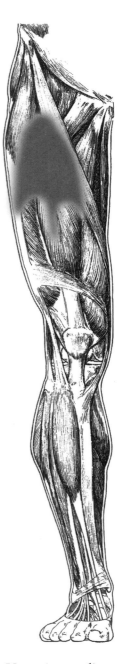

Rectus femoris   *Vastus lateralis*   *Vastus medialis*   *Vastus intermedius*

Quadriceps pain pattern

Constrictions in rectus femoris must be reduced before an attempt is made to identify and reduce constrictions in vastus intermedius. Once rectus femoris is free of constriction, taut bands may be located in vastus intermedius by locating the proximal lateral border of rectus femoris. Follow this border distally until the fingers can palpate vastus intermedius, deep to rectus femoris, close to the femur.

Pain pattern: Pain from active trigger points is experienced at various locations relative to the muscle most involved. *Rectus femoris:* Pain is experienced in the anterior knee, sometimes deep in the joint. Pain may be experienced at night; walking down stairs may be difficult. *Vastus lateralis:* Pain is referred to the posterolateral aspect of the knee; it can refer throughout the full course of the lateral thigh to the knee and as high as the crest of the ilium. Distal trigger points may immobilize the patella, causing pain while walking. Symptoms may include difficulty lying on the same side at night. *Vastus medialis:* Anteromedial knee pain; pain extends through the distal one-half of the medial thigh; buckling of the knee. *Vastus intermedius:* Pain is referred over the anterior thigh, extending anterolaterally over the upper thigh. Pain may be most intense at midthigh level. Walking up stairs may be difficult, as is straightening the leg after sitting.

Causative or perpetuating factors: Sudden overload through misstep or fall; sustained overload due to excessively tightened hamstring muscles.

Satellite trigger points: Each muscle of the quadriceps group may develop satellite trigger points in response to the presence of trigger points in any other muscle of the group. Additional satellite trigger points could also appear in semimembranosus, semitendinosus, biceps femoris, tensor fasciae latae, and iliopsoas.

Affected organ systems: *Rectus femoris, vastus lateralis, and vastus intermedius:* digestive system. *Vastus medialis:* genitourinary and reproductive systems.

Associated zones, meridians, and points: *Rectus femoris:* ventral zone; Foot Yang Ming Stomach meridian; ST 31–34, SP 10 and 11. *Vastus lateralis:* ventral and lateral zones; Foot Yang Ming Stomach meridian, Foot Shao Yang Gall Bladder meridian; ST 31–34, GB 31. *Vastus medialis:* ventral zone; Foot Tai Yin Spleen meridian; SP 10 and 11. *Vastus intermedius:* ventral zone; Foot Yang Ming Stomach meridian; ST 31–34, SP 10 and 11.

Stretch exercise: Stand, or sit on the edge of a chair. Flex the lower leg and grasp the ankle with the homolateral hand. Lift the heel toward the buttock and extend the thigh and hip as far backward as possible. Tilt the pelvis to avoid excessive arching of the lumbar spine. Hold this position for a count of ten to fifteen.

Strengthening exercise: Sit on a chair with the feet on the floor. Fully extend the working leg to a count of two. Return the leg to the starting position to a count of four. Repeat this exercise ten to twelve times, working one leg at a time.

Ankle weights may be used to increase the demand placed on the quadriceps during this exercise. The amount of weight used must be gauged according to the needs and capabilities of the patient.

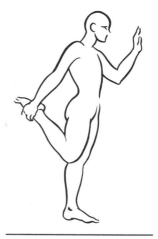

Stretch exercise: Quadriceps

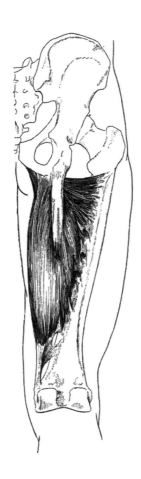 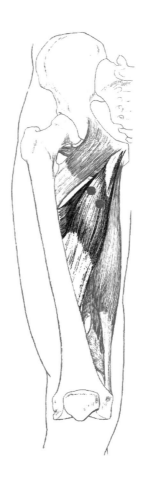

Adductor magnus   *Adductor longus*
                          and Adductor brevis

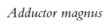

Adductors and trigger points

ADDUCTORS

ADDUCTOR MAGNUS, ADDUCTOR LONGUS, ADDUCTOR BREVIS

Proximal attachment: *Adductor magnus:* inferior pubic ramus, ramus of ischium, ischial tuberosity. *Adductor longus:* pubic tubercle. *Adductor brevis:* inferior ramus of the pubis.

Distal attachment: *Adductor magnus:* linea aspera of the posterior femur, adductor tubercle of the medial femur. *Adductor longus:* linea aspera on the middle one-third of the femur. *Adductor brevis:* proximal aspect of the linea aspera of the femur, lateral and deep to adductor longus.

Action: *Adductor magnus:* anterior fibers adduct and internally rotate the thigh; posterior fibers extend the thigh. *Adductor longus and adductor brevis:* adduction of the thigh at the hip.

Palpation: Of the muscles in the adductor group, adductor longus is the most prominent and most readily accessible to palpation.

To locate the adductors, identify the following structures:

- Femoral triangle—Bounded superiorly by the inguinal ligament, medially by adductor longus, and laterally by sartorius. The floor of the femoral triangle is formed medially by pectinius and laterally by iliopsoas. Within this triangle the femoral pulse can be palpated 2 to 3 centimeters (approximately 1 inch) inferior to the inguinal ligament, at the midline of the base of the triangle which it forms. Both the femoral artery and femoral lymph glands lie superficial to iliopsoas and pectinius, which themselves lie superficial to the hip joint. The femoral artery lies just superficial to

the head of the femur. The pulse point of the femoral artery can be palpated just superficial to the head of the femur, inferior to the midpoint of the inguinal ligament.

- Ischial tuberosity—Easily palpable when seated, this bony prominence carries most of the weight of the torso in the seated position. It is located at the center of the buttock, approximately level with the gluteal fold.

Palpate adductor magnus and adductor longus with the patient lying supine. To palpate adductor magnus, flex the leg of the thigh to be palpated, then externally rotate and abduct the thigh in order to position the sole of the foot of that leg approximately 8 to 10 inches lateral to the inner thigh of the extended leg. If necessary, a pillow may be placed beneath the bent knee for patient comfort. Palpate adductor magnus posterior to adductor longus and adductor brevis, from the ischial tuberosity to the medial aspect of the femur.

To palpate adductor longus, place the sole of the foot against the inner thigh of the extended leg. In this position adductor longus becomes clearly visible and palpable. Palpate adductor longus anterior to adductor magnus, from its proximal aspect near the pubis to its distal aspect at the middle one-third of the femur.

Adductor longus and pectineus lie superficial to adductor brevis. Therefore adductor brevis cannot be directly palpated.

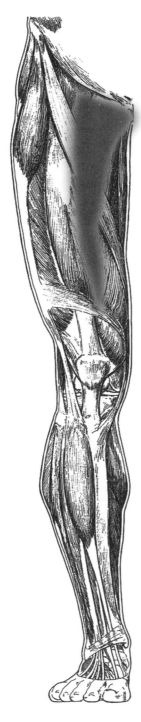

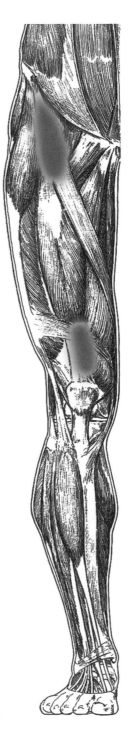

Adductor magnus

Adductor longus
and Adductor brevis

—————————

Adductors pain pattern

Pain pattern: *Adductor magnus:* Trigger points in the proximal aspect of the muscle, near the ischial tuberosity, refer severe, deep pelvic pain that may include pain at the pubic bone, vagina, rectum, and possibly the bladder. Trigger points in the middle portion of adductor magnus refer pain to the anteromedial aspect of the thigh, from the groin to just above the knee. *Adductor longus and adductor brevis:* Pain in the groin that is experienced during activity; reduced abduction and external rotation of the thigh. Pain deep in the groin and possibly the anteromedial aspect of the upper thigh; pain above the medial aspect of the knee and possibly over the shin. Trigger points near the proximal attachment of adductor longus may cause knee pain and stiffness.

Causative or perpetuating factors: Sudden overload due to a misstep or fall; arthritis of the hip joint; sustained overload due to activities such as horseback riding or sitting with the legs crossed for lengthy periods of time; emotional stresses.

Satellite trigger points: Each muscle of the adductor group may develop satellite trigger points in response to the presence of trigger points in any other muscle of the group. Additional satellite trigger points could also appear in vastus medialis and gracilis.

Affected organ system: Reproductive system.

Associated zones, meridians, and points: *Adductor magnus:* Ventral zone; Foot Jue Yin Liver meridian, Foot Shao Yin Kidney meridian; LIV 10 and 11, BL 36 and 37. *Adductor longus and adductor brevis:* ventral zone, Foot Jue Yin Liver meridian; LIV 9, 10, and 11.

Stretch exercises: Adductor magnus forms a functional hamstring with the short head of the biceps femoris. Therapeutic stretching of the adductor group must therefore coincide with therapeutic stretching of the hamstring group in order to obtain the full benefit for each muscle group.

1. Lying with the buttocks against a wall and the legs extended upward on the wall, slowly separate the legs to stretch the inner thighs. Hold this position for 30 to 60 seconds, allowing gravity to act on the abducted legs.

2. Positioned supine, with the thigh and leg of the affected side off the side of an examining table or bed, flex the thigh and leg of the unaffected side to fix the pelvis, keeping the lumbar spine flat on the table. Abduct the thigh and leg, allowing it to hang off the side of the table or bed. The force of gravity will stretch the upper groin region. Hold this position for a count of 20 to 30.

Strengthening exercise: Sitting on the edge of a chair, place a large, soft ball between the thighs. Adduct the thighs, squeezing the ball. Hold for a count of five to eight and release. Repeat ten to twelve times.

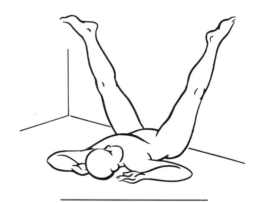

Stretch exercise 1: Adductors

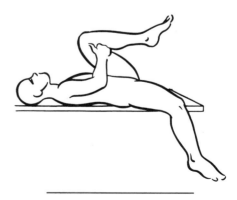

Stretch exercise 2: Adductors

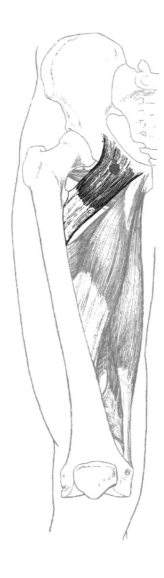

Pectineus and trigger point

PECTINEUS

Proximal attachment: Crest of the superior ramus of the pubis.

Distal attachment: On the femur, just distal to the lesser trochanter.

Action: Flexion, adduction, and internal rotation of the thigh at the hip.

Palpation: To locate pectineus, identify the following structures:

- Femoral triangle—Bounded superiorly by the inguinal ligament, medially by adductor longus (see muscle description on page 181) and laterally by sartorius (see muscle description on page 191). The floor of the femoral triangle is formed medially by pectineus and laterally by iliopsoas. Within this triangle the femoral pulse can be palpated 2 to 3 centimeters (approximately 1 inch) inferior to the inguinal ligament, at the midline of the base of the triangle that it forms. Both the femoral artery and femoral lymph glands lie superficial to iliopsoas and pectinius, which themselves lie superficial to the hip joint. The femoral artery lies just superficial to the head of the femur. The pulse point of the femoral artery can be palpatated just superficial to the head of the femur, inferior to the midpoint of the inguinal ligament.

- Pubic tubercle—The bony prominence at the lateral aspect of the pubic crest. The pubic tubercle serves as the distal attachment for the inguinal ligament.

Palpate pectineus with the patient lying supine. Abduct and externally rotate the thigh to be palpated, then flex the leg to bring the sole of the foot adjacent to the opposite inner thigh. If necessary a pillow may be placed beneath the bent knee for patient comfort. Locate the femoral triangle and pubic tubercle. Pectineus occupies the medial aspect of the floor of the femoral triangle. To locate pectineus palpate within the femoral triangle, approximately 1 inch lateral and 1 inch distal to the pubic tubercle.

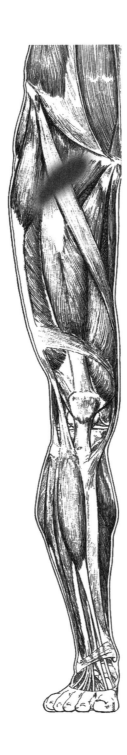

Pectineus pain pattern

Pain pattern: Deep, local groin pain, just distal to the inguinal ligament.

Causative or perpetuating factors: Sudden overload from an unexpected fall; chronic overload in adduction and flexion, such as sitting cross-legged for an extended period of time; diseases or surgeries affecting the hip joint.

Satellite trigger points: Adductor longus, adductor brevis, adductor magnus, iliopsoas.

Affected organ system: Reproductive system.

Associated zones, meridians, and points: Ventral zone; Foot Jue Yin Liver meridian; LIV 9, 10, and 11.

Stretch exercise: Lying on a table or bed, abduct the affected thigh and leg and allow the limb to hang off the side of the table or bed. Flex the unaffected thigh and leg to fix the pelvis, keeping the lumbar spine flat on the table or bed. Let gravity stretch the upper groin region. Hold for a count of twenty to thirty.

Strengthening exercise: Sitting on the edge of a chair, place a large, soft ball between the thighs. Adduct the thighs, squeezing the ball. Hold for a count of five to eight, and release. Repeat ten to twelve times.

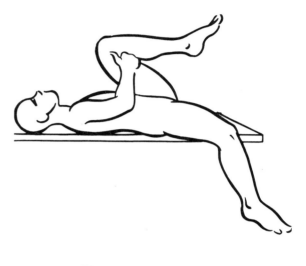

Stretch exercise: Pectineus

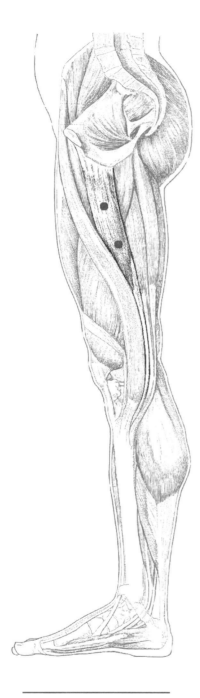

Gracilis and trigger points

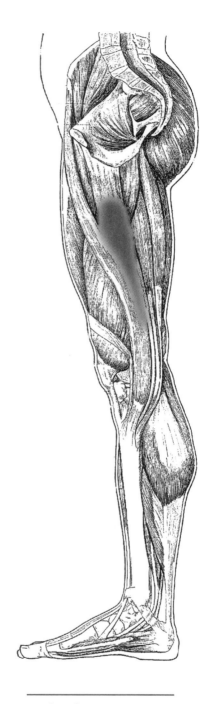

Gracilis pain pattern

GRACILIS

Proximal attachment: Inferior pubic ramus.

Distal attachment: Medial side of the superior part of the tibia, distal to the tibial condyle, forming the pes anserinus with sartorius and semitendinosus.

Action: Adduction of the thigh at the hip; flexion of the leg; assists in internal rotation of the thigh and flexed leg.

Palpation: To locate gracilis, identify the following structures:

- Medial surface of the tibial condyle
- Distal attachment of semitendinosus—Identify the popliteal fossa, the posterior aspect of the knee joint that appears as a hollow when the knee is flexed. The distal attachment of semitendinosus forms the medial border of the popliteal fossa; the lateral border is formed by the tendon of biceps femoris.

Palpate the knee of the flexed leg at the popliteal region and identify the prominent tendon of semitendinosus forming the medial border of the popliteal fossa. Move slightly medially to locate the tendon of gracilis, which lies anterior and medial to the tendon of semitendinosus. Offering resistance to internal rotation of the thigh allows gracilis to become more prominent. Palpate this thin, bandlike muscle along its course on the medial aspect of the thigh.

Pain pattern: Hot, stinging, superficial pain along the medial thigh.

Causative or perpetuating factors: Sudden overload due to a misstep or fall; arthritis of the hip joint; sustained overload due to activities such as horseback riding or sitting with the legs crossed for lengthy periods of time; emotional stresses.

Satellite trigger points: Sartorius.

Affected organ systems: Reproductive and genitourinary systems.

Associated zones, meridians, and points: Ventral zone; Foot Jue Yin Liver meridian; SP 9, LIV 8–11.

Stretch exercise: Lying with the buttocks against a wall and the legs extended upward on the wall, slowly separate the legs to stretch the inner thighs. Hold this position for 30 to 60 seconds, allowing gravity to act on the abducted legs.

Strengthening exercise: Sitting on the edge of a chair, place a large, soft ball between the thighs. Adduct the thighs, squeezing the ball. Hold for a count of five to eight, and release. Repeat ten to twelve times.

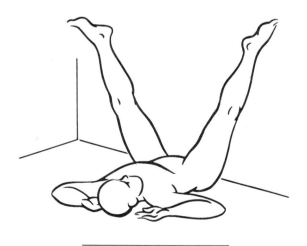

Stretch exercise: Gracilis

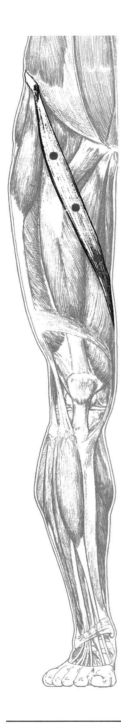

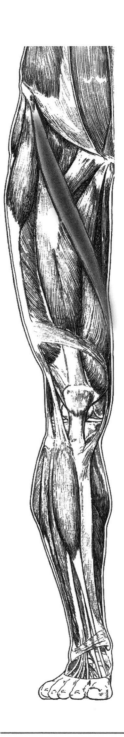

Sartorius and trigger points

Sartorius pain pattern

Sartorius

Proximal attachment: Anterior superior iliac spine (ASIS).

Distal attachment: Medial side of the superior part of the tibia, distal to the tibial condyle, forming the pes anserinus with semitendinosus and gracilis.

Action: Assists in flexion, abduction, and external rotation of the thigh; assists in hip flexion and knee flexion during walking.

Palpation: To locate sartorius, identify the following structures:

- Anterior superior iliac spine (ASIS)—Anterior bony projection lying somewhat below the iliac crest, readily palpable. The ASIS serves as the proximal attachment of the inguinal ligament.
- Medial surface of the tibial condyle
- Distal attachment of semitendinosus—Identify the popliteal fossa, the posterior aspect of the knee joint that appears as a hollow when the knee is flexed. The distal attachment of semitendinosus forms the medial border of the popliteal fossa; the lateral border is formed by the tendon of biceps femoris.

Locate sartorius with the patient seated and the leg flexed to 90 degrees. Offering resistance to external rotation of the thigh, sartorius will become prominent from its attachment at the ASIS. Palpate sartorius from the ASIS throughout its course to its distal attachment, distal to the medial surface of the tibial condyle. The tendon of insertion of sartorius lies anterior to the tendons of insertion of gracilis and semitendinosus and forms the flattest and most anterior tendon of the pes anserinus.

Pain pattern: Superficial tingling pain along the course of the muscle.

Causative or perpetuating factors: Trigger points occur in this muscle as a result of its placement within the pain referral zone of an associated muscle.

Satellite trigger points: Rectus femoris, vastus lateralis, vastus medialis, vastus intermedius.

Affected organ system: Genitourinary system.

Associated zones, meridians, and points: Ventral zone; Foot Yang Ming Stomach meridian; ST 31, LIV 8.

Stretch exercise: Digital compressions directly along the muscle produce an effective local stretch.

Strengthening exercise: Strengthening exercises specific to this muscle are generally not indicated.

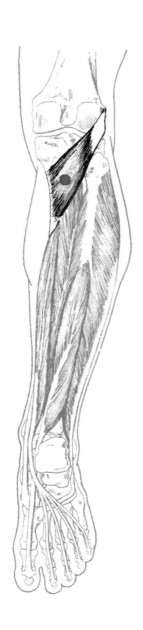

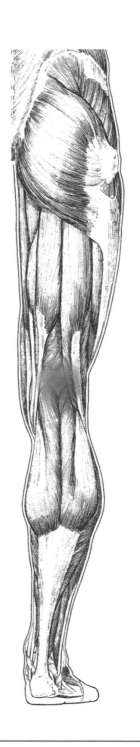

Popliteus and trigger point

Popliteus pain pattern

POPLITEUS

Proximal attachment: Lateral aspect of the lateral condyle of the femur.

Distal attachment: Proximal one-third of the posterior aspect of the tibia.

Action: Internally rotates the leg on the femur when the thigh is fixed and the leg is free and externally rotates the femur on the leg in weight bearing when the leg is fixed; unlocks the knee joint to facilitate bending of the knee; prevents forward displacement of the femur on the tibia when crouching.

Palpation: Popliteus forms part of the distal aspect of the floor of the popliteal fossa. Palpate popliteus with the patient side-lying on the affected side, the leg slightly flexed. The distal, medial attachment of the muscle lies on the posterior aspect of the tibia and can be palpated between the tendon of semitendinosus and the medial head of gastrocnemius. To palpate taut bands within this aspect of popliteus, laterally displace the overlying gastrocnemius and soleus. The proximal, lateral end of popliteus lies in the popliteal space just above the head of the fibula, between the tendon of biceps femoris and the lateral head of gastrocnemius and plantaris. Palpate through the overlying musculature.

Pain pattern: Pain in the back of the knee, often when crouching, running, or walking downhill or going down stairs; inability to straighten the knee fully without pain. Pain from trigger points in this muscle is rarely experienced in isolation; pain is most often experienced in combination with gastrocnemius and biceps femoris, which are usually identified as the source of the posterior knee pain. Once the gastrocnemius and biceps femoris trigger points are reduced, popliteus can be more readily identified as the source of posterior knee pain.

Causative or perpetuating factors: Muscle overload while braking the forward motion of the femur during a twisting turn, with the body weight on the slightly bent knee of the side to which the body is turning. This is especially common in soccer or football or when running or skiing downhill. Trigger points in popliteus may develop secondary to a tear of the plantaris muscle and may remain long after the plantaris tear is healed.

Satellite trigger points: Gastrocnemius.

Affected organ systems: Genitourinary system.

Associated zones, meridians, and points: Dorsal zone; Foot Tai Yang Bladder meridian; BL 39 and 40.

Stretch exercises: Flex the leg 15 to 20 degrees; with the thigh fixed, laterally rotate the leg. Make sure that the leg (not the thigh) is being rotated. Hold the position for a count of fifteen to twenty. Repeat two to three times.

Strengthening exercise: Due to the nature of this muscle, strengthening exercises are not necessary.

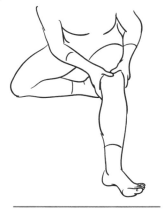

Stretch exercise: Popliteus

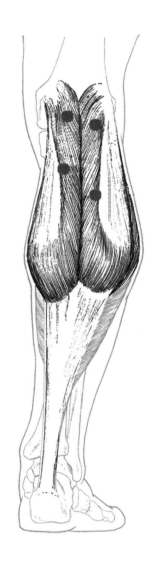

Gastrocnemius and trigger points

GASTROCNEMIUS

Proximal attachment: By two heads, the medial head attaching to the medial epicondyle of the femur, the lateral head attaching to the lateral epicondyle of the femur.

Distal attachment: Via the tendocalcaneus (Achilles tendon) to the posterior surface of the calcaneus, with soleus.

Action: Plantar flexion; aids in flexion of the knee when the leg is not bearing weight.

Palpation: To locate gastrocnemius, identify the following structures:

- Medial epicondyle of the femur
- Lateral epicondyle of the femur

- Tendocalcaneus (Achilles tendon)—The thickest and strongest tendon in the body, the tendocalcaneus is the common tendon of insertion for the gastrocnemius and soleus muscles. This tendon is palpable from the lower one-third of the calf to the calcaneus.

Due to its superficial position on the posterior calf, gastrocnemius is easily palpable. Palpate both the medial and lateral heads throughout their course, to their attachment to the tendocalcaneus. Note that the medial head is somewhat longer than the lateral head.

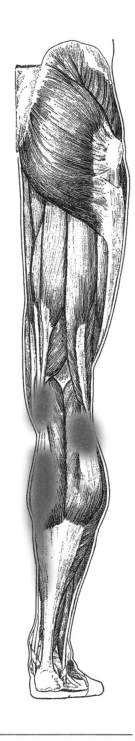

Gastrocnemius pain pattern

Pain pattern: Local calf pain without reduced range of motion or weakness; pain in the back of the knee; possibly pain in the instep; nocturnal calf cramps.

Causative or perpetuating factors: Chronic overload due to excessive plantar flexion; immobility of the legs; reduced circulation into the legs.

Satellite trigger points: Soleus, hamstrings.

Affected organ system: Genitourinary system.

Associated zones, meridians, and points: Dorsal zone; Foot Tai Yang Bladder meridian; BL 56, 57, and 58, GB 36.

Stretch exercises:

1. Place the ball of the foot on a step or curb and allow the heel of the foot to drop below the level of the step. Keep the knee straight as you stretch the calf. Hold this position for a count of twenty-five to thirty.

2. Stand approximately 12 inches from a wall, the hands placed on the wall at the chest level. Place the leg to be stretched approximately 18 inches behind the other, keeping the toes of both feet facing the wall and the feet hip-width apart. Bend the front knee, keeping the rear leg straight. Hold this position for a count of twenty-five to thirty.

Strengthening exercise: Standing and holding on to a wall or chair for balance, raise up onto the ball of the foot, bringing the heel well off the floor. Hold this position for a count of five. Slowly return the heel to the floor. Repeat ten to twelve times.

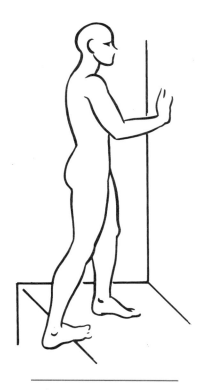

Stretch exercise 1: Gastrocnemius

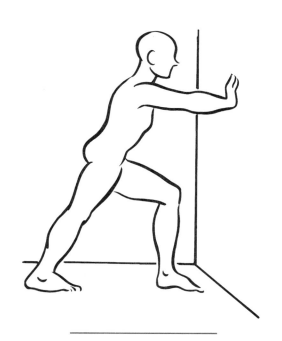

Stretch exercise 2: Gastrocnemius

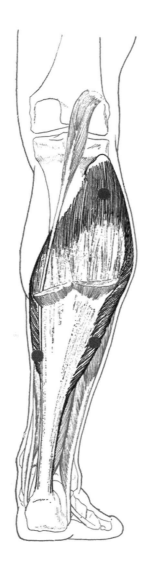

Soleus and trigger points

SOLEUS

Proximal attachment: Posterior aspect of the head of the fibula and the proximal one-third of the posterior fibula and middle one-third of the tibia.

Distal attachment: Via the tendocalcaneus (Achilles tendon) to the posterior surface of the calcaneus, with gastrocnemius.

Action: Plantar flexion of the foot; assists inversion; contributes to knee stability; provides ankle stability.

Palpation: To identify soleus, locate the following structures:

- Tendocalcaneus (Achilles tendon)—The thickest and strongest tendon in the body, the tendocalcaneus is the common tendon of insertion for the gastrocnemius and soleus muscles. This tendon is palpable from the lower one-third of the calf to the calcaneus.

Soleus lies deep to gastrocnemius. Palpate soleus on the distal one-half of the lower leg, lateral and distal to the lateral head of gastrocnemius and medial and distal to the medial head of gastrocnemius.

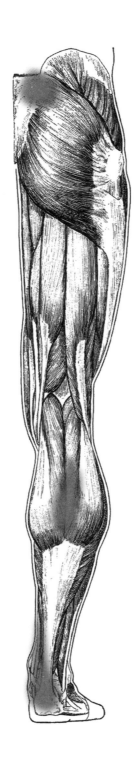

Soleus pain pattern

Pain pattern: Heel pain, tenderness, restricted dorsiflexion; walking uphill or up stairs may be difficult. Trigger points in the proximal aspect of the muscle radiate to the posterior calf; distal trigger points radiate to the posterior aspect of the heel, possibly including its plantar surface and the distal aspect of the Achilles tendon; pain may be experienced at the sacroiliac joint on the same side.

Causative or perpetuating factors: Chronic overload due to excessive plantar flexion; sudden overload due to misstep; poor circulation in the legs.

Satellite trigger points: Gastrocnemius, homolateral quadriceps.

Affected organ system: Cardiovascular system.

Associated zones, meridians, and points: Dorsal zone; Foot Tai Yang Bladder meridian, Foot Shao Yin Kidney meridian; BL 59, KI 7, KI 9.

Stretch exercises:

1. Place the ball of the foot on a step or curb and allow the heel of the foot to drop below the level of the step. Keep the knee bent as you stretch the calf. Hold this position for a count of twenty-five to thirty.

2. Stand approximately 12 inches away from a wall, the hands placed on the wall at chest level. Place the leg to be stretched approximately 18 inches behind the other, keeping the toes of both feet facing the wall and the feet hip-width apart. Bend both knees to stretch soleus. Hold this position for a count of twenty-five to thirty.

Strengthening exercise: Standing and holding on to a wall or chair for balance, raise up onto the ball of the foot, bringing the heel well off the floor. Hold this position for a count of five. Slowly return the heel to the floor. Repeat ten to twelve times.

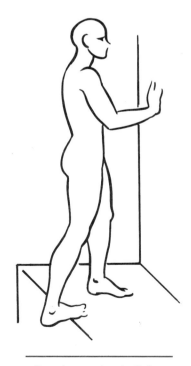

Stretch exercise 1: Soleus

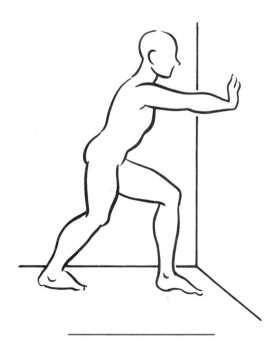

Stretch exercise 2: Soleus

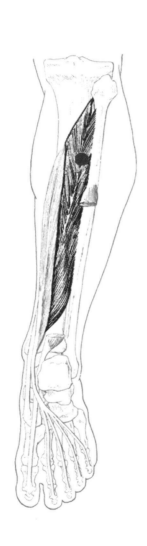

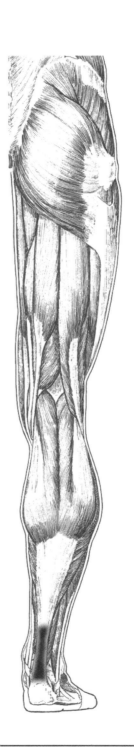

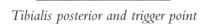

Tibialis posterior and trigger point

Tibialis posterior pain pattern

TIBIALIS POSTERIOR

Proximal attachment: Proximal two-thirds of the posterior surfaces of the tibia and the fibula and the interosseus membrane.

Distal attachment: Passing behind the medial malleolus to attach to most of the bones that form the arch of the foot: the navicular, each cuneiform, and the cuboid; the calcaneus; and metatarsals 2, 3, and 4.

Action: Inverts and adducts (supinates) the free foot; assists in plantar flexion. Prevents excessive pronation of the foot during walking; prevents excessive weight bearing on the medial foot; distributes weight evenly along the heads of the metatarsals, helping to shift the weight laterally.

Palpation: Tibialis posterior is the deepest muscle of the calf, lying between the interosseus membrane anteriorly and the soleus posteriorly. Along with flexor digitorum longus and flexor hallucis longus it comprises the deep posterior compartment of the leg. Due to the depth of its placement on the leg this muscle cannot be palpated directly; however, tenderness can be elicited through deep palpation. Identify the posterior border of the tibia on the posteromedial surface of the leg. Palpate the proximal half of the lower leg, partially displacing the soleus posteriorly, to identify the posterior surface of the tibia through the overlying soleus.

Pain pattern: Tibialis posterior is rarely involved in isolation from other calf muscles. Pain radiates over the Achilles tendon above the heel; additional pain may cover the mid-calf, the heel, and the plantar surface of the foot and toes. Pain is experienced in the sole of the foot when walking or running, particularly on uneven surfaces.

Causative or perpetuating factors: Jogging on uneven surfaces such as crowned roads; hypermobility of the midfoot; badly worn footwear that does not protect against eversion and rocking of the foot.

Satellite trigger points: Flexor digitorum longus, flexor hallucis longus, and the peroneal muscles.

Affected organ systems: Genitourinary system.

Associated zones, meridians, and points: Dorsal zone; Foot Tai Yang Bladder meridian; BL 55, 56, and 57.

Stretch exercise: Stretch this muscle by dorsiflexing and everting the foot. Sitting with the legs extended in front of you, place a belt or towel around the midfoot of the leg to be stretched. Pull the band toward you, stretching the posterior calf. Pull with slightly greater force on the outside of the foot, which will allow the lateral side of the foot to be everted. Hold this position for a count of fifteen to twenty. Repeat three to five times.

Strengthening exercise: Due to the nature of this muscle, strengthening exercises are generally not necessary.

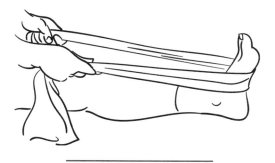

Stretch exercise: Tibialis posterior

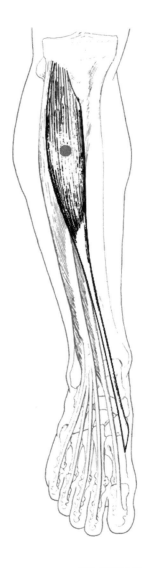

Tibialis anterior and trigger point

TIBIALIS ANTERIOR

Proximal attachment: Lateral condyle of the tibia and the upper one-half to two-thirds of the lateral surface of the body of the tibia, interosseus membrane, and surrounding fascia.

Distal attachment: Medial and plantar surfaces of the medial cuneiform bone and the base of the first metatarsal.

Action: Dorsiflexion and supination (inversion) of the foot. Helps to maintain standing balance, prevents foot slap at heel strike, and helps foot clear floor at swing phase. Vigorously active during most sports activities, including jogging, running, sprinting, and two-legged jumps. Helps maintain standing balance.

Palpation: Tibialis anterior, peroneus tertius, extensor digitorum longus, and extensor hallucis longus comprise the anterior compartment of the leg. This superficial calf muscle can be palpated at the proximal one-half to two-thirds of the lateral calf. Palpate the muscle mass lateral to the sharp edge of the shin, from the lateral condyle of the tibia distally toward the ankle. Continue palpating the muscle as it crosses the ankle medially and attaches at the medial arch. The muscle can be visually identified at the level of the ankle joint by dorsiflexing and inverting the foot. Trigger points are commonly located at the junction of the proximal and middle thirds of the tibia; however, they can develop in the midbelly of the muscle at any level.

Pain pattern: Pain at the anteromedial ankle and the great toe. Some pain may be experienced along the course of the shin to the ankle. Symptoms associated with trigger points may include ankle weakness, tripping or falling when walking because of weak dorsiflexion, and foot drop.

Causative or perpetuating factors: Muscle overload that may occur secondary to ankle sprain or fracture; walking on rough ground or slanted surfaces; excessive tightness in the triceps surae.

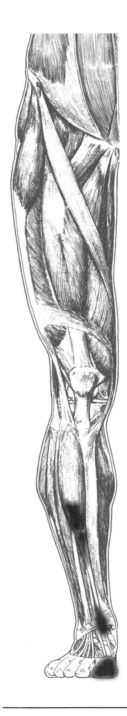

Tibialis anterior pain pattern

Satellite trigger points: Peroneus longus, extensor hallucis longus, possibly extensor digitorum longus.

Affected organ systems: Digestive system.

Associated zones, meridians, and points: Lateral zone; Foot Yang Ming Stomach meridian; ST 36–40; LIV 4.

Stretch exercise: Stretch the tibialis anterior by crossing a strongly pointed foot over the ankle of the standing leg. Bend the knee of the standing leg into the back of the knee of the bent leg. Care should be taken to ensure that the heel is raised and that the ankle is neither supinated nor pronated.

Strengthening exercise: Stretch a dynaband or other elastic exercise band between the legs of a chair or table 3 to 4 inches from the floor. Sit on the floor with the legs extended and position the foot so the band lies across the dorsum of the foot (not across the toes). Flex and supinate (invert) the foot against the resistance provided by the band. Hold for a count of three to five. Repeat five to ten times.

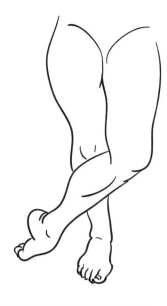

Stretch exercise: Tibialis anterior

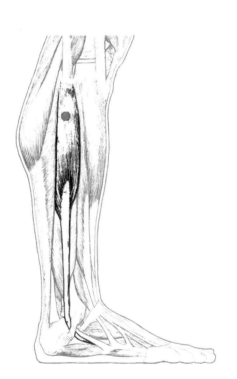

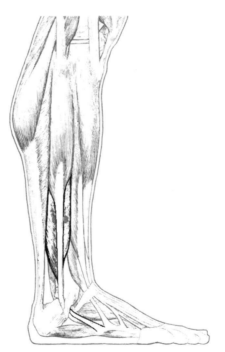

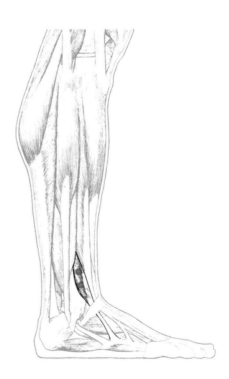

Peroneus longus   *Peroneus brevis*   *Peroneus tertius*

Peroneals and trigger points

PERONEAL MUSCLES

PERONEUS LONGUS, PERONEUS BREVIS, PERONEUS TERTIUS

Proximal attachment: *Peroneus longus:* head of the fibula and upper two-thirds of the lateral surface of the fibula and the adjacent intermuscular septa. *Peroneus brevis:* lying deep to longus, distal two-thirds of the lateral surface of the fibula and the adjacent intermuscular septa. *Peroneus tertius:* distal one-half of the anterior margin of the fibula and the adjacent intermuscular septum, in common with the lower fibers of extensor digitorum longus.

Distal attachment: *Peroneus longus:* passing behind the lateral malleolus, running obliquely across the sole of the foot from lateral to medial, and ending on the base of the first metatarsal and the medial cuneiform bones. *Peroneus brevis:* passing behind the lateral malleolus, ending at the dorsal surface of the base of the fifth metatarsal. *Peroneus tertius:* passing in front of the lateral malleolus, ending on the dorsal surface of the base of the fifth metatarsal.

Action: *Peroneus longus and peroneus brevis:* eversion and weak plantar flexion of the foot; controls excessive inversion and mediolateral balance in walking. *Peroneus tertius:* dorsiflexion and eversion of the foot. As a group the peroneals are prime movers in the eversion of the free foot, working with extensor digitorum longus.

Palpation: Peroneus longus and peroneus brevis comprise the lateral compartment of the leg. Peroneus tertius, along with tibialis anterior, extensor digitorum longus, and extensor hallucis longus, comprise the anterior compartment of the leg. To palpate the peroneals, first identify the head and shaft of the fibula and the extensor digitorum longus, which lies just anterior to peroneus longus. Peroneus longus taut bands can be easily identified against the shaft of the fibula. Trigger points in peroneus longus are most commonly found approximately 1 inch distal to the head of the fibula.

For peroneus brevis, palpate along the shaft of the fibula on either side of longus, near the junction of the middle and lower thirds of the leg. Unlike longus and brevis, peroneus tertius lies proximal and anterior to the lateral malleolus. Palpate fibers of peroneus tertius distal and anterior to brevis. The tendon of peroneus tertius is readily palpable and observable in the anterolateral aspect of the foot, lateral to the extensor digitorum longus tendon, when the patient everts the foot.

Pain pattern: For peroneus longus and brevis, the pain pattern is over the lateral malleolus: above, behind, and below it and possibly along the lateral aspect of the foot. For peroneus tertius, the pain pattern is over the anterolateral aspect of the ankle, anterior to the lateral malleolus, with some pain on the outer side of the heel. Symptoms include weak or unstable ankles; there are complaints of pain and tenderness in the ankle over the lateral malleolus, particularly after an inversion sprain. Tenderness due to trigger points can be differentiated from a lateral ligament injury by the absence of swelling in the immediate area and the presence of pain in a larger, more diffuse area.

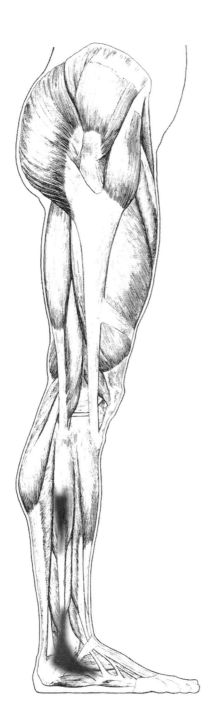

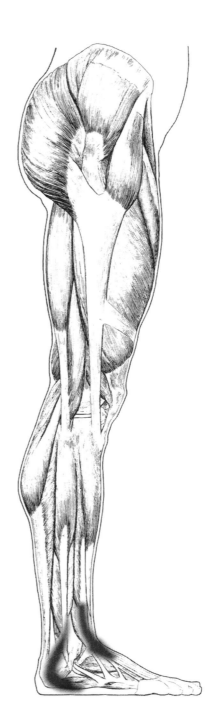

Peroneus longus and Peroneus brevis

Peroneus tertius

Peroneals pain pattern

Causative or perpetuating factors: Ankle inversion or twisting; prolonged immobilization of the leg and foot by a cast; chronic tightness of the tibialis anterior or tibialis posterior; crossing legs when seated, wearing high heels; tight elastic around the leg; flat feet; sleeping with the feet strongly plantar flexed; as satellite trigger points from trigger points existing in anterior fibers of gluteus minimus.

Satellite trigger points: Peroneus longus, peroneus brevis, peroneus tertius, extensor digitorum longus, tibialis anterior, tibialis posterior, extensor hallucis longus, flexor hallucis longus.

Affected organ systems: Gastrointestinal system.

Associated zones, meridians, and points: Lateral zone; Foot Shao Yang Gall Bladder meridian; GB 37–40.

Stretch exercise: Sit with the leg to be stretched extended in front of you. Place a strap or towel around the foot. Holding the towel, pull the foot gently, allowing it to move into dorsiflexion, inversion, and adduction. Hold the position for a count of fifteen to twenty. Repeat three to five times.

Strengthening exercise: Due to the nature of this muscle, strengthening exercises are generally not necessary.

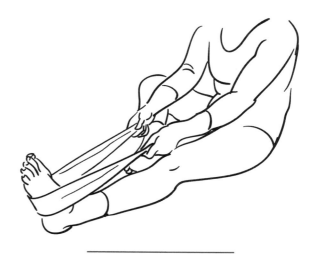

Stretch exercise: Peroneals

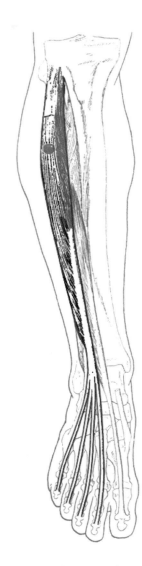

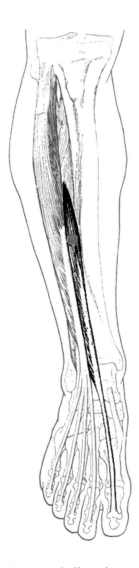

Extensor digitorum longus　　　　*Extensor hallucis longus*

Long extensors of the toes and trigger points

Long Extensors of the Toes

Extensor Digitorum Longus and Extensor Hallucis Longus

Proximal attachment: *Extensor digitorum longus:* lateral condyle of the tibia, proximal three-quarters of the fibula, interosseus membrane. *Extensor hallucis longus:* middle one-third of the anterior surface of the fibula, interosseus membrane.

Distal attachment: *Extensor digitorum longus:* middle and distal phalanges of the four lateral toes. *Extensor hallucis longus:* distal phalange of the great toe.

Action: *Extensor digitorum longus:* extension of the four lateral toes; assists in dorsiflexion and eversion of the foot; works very strongly in a vertical jump from a standing position. *Extensor digitorum longus:* extension of the great toe; assists in dorsiflexion and inversion of the foot.

Palpation: Extensor digitorum longus and extensor hallucis longus, along with tibialis anterior and peroneus tertius, comprise the anterior compartment of the leg.

To palpate extensor digitorum longus, identify tibialis anterior anteriorly and peroneus longus posteriorly to locate extensor digitorum longus. Palpate taut bands approximately 3 inches distal to the head of the fibula. Extensor hallucis longus lies between and deep to tibialis anterior and extensor digitorum longus throughout the upper two-thirds of the lower leg. It can be palpated where it becomes superficial just distal to the level of the lower one-third of the leg, anterior to the fibula.

Pain pattern: *Extensor digitorum longus:* Pain on the dorsum of the foot and the central three digits. Sometimes pain can be experienced at the ankle; the pain may move upward as far as the lower one-half of the lower leg. *Extensor hallucis longus:* Pain at the first metatarsal and the great toe. It may also extend toward the ankle, following the course of the muscle. Symptoms include pain on the dorsum of the foot, "foot slap" during walking, and night cramps along the course of the muscle. Presence of taut bands and trigger points over time may lead to the development of hammertoes or claw toes.

Causative or perpetuating factors: L4-L5 radiculopathy; acute stress overload caused by walking in soft sand; walking or jogging on uneven ground or crowned roads; tripping or falling; using the lengthened muscle in continual plantar flexion position (such as wearing high-heeled shoes or driving with a steep accelerator pedal); prolonged plantar flexion; prolonged immobilization as a result of wearing a cast; very tight gastrocnemius and soleus muscles.

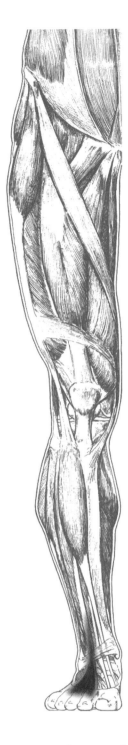

Extensor digitorum longus

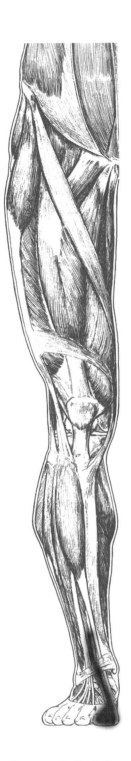

Extensor hallucis longus

Long extensors of the toes pain pattern

Satellite trigger points: Peroneus longus, peroneus brevis, peroneus tertius, tibialis anterior.

Affected organ systems: Digestive system.

Associated zones, meridians, and points: Lateral zone; Foot Yang Ming Stomach meridian; ST 40 and 41.

Stretch exercise: Position a strongly pointed foot over the ankle of the standing leg, placing the toes of the leg to be stretched beside the heel of the standing leg. Bend the knee of the standing leg into the back of the knee of the bent leg to stretch the dorsum of the foot.

Strengthening exercise: Work the extensors by alternating plantar flexion and dorsiflexion of the foot and toes. Begin with your legs extended in front of you and your foot and ankle in a neutral, relaxed position. Plantarflex the foot and toes strongly. Hold for a count of three to five. Beginning with the toes, slowly extend the toes and dorsiflex the foot. Hold for a count of three to five. Repeat these two actions five to seven times, moving through each position slowly and without allowing the foot to evert or invert.

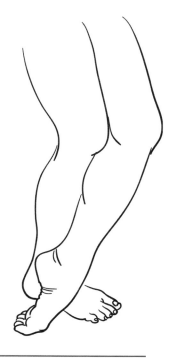

Stretch exercise: Long extensors of the toes

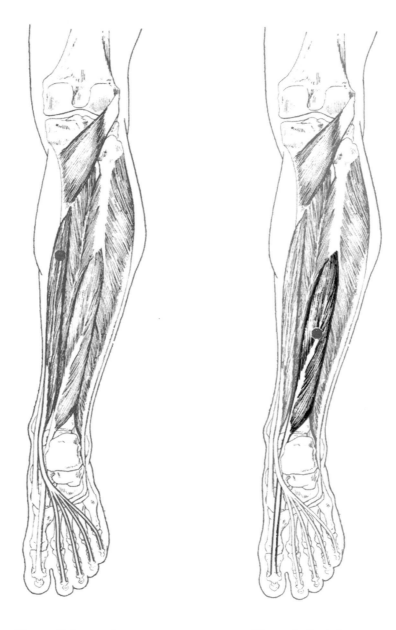

Flexor digitorum longus   *Flexor hallucis longus*

———————————

Long flexors of the toes and trigger points

LONG FLEXORS OF THE TOES

FLEXOR DIGITORUM LONGUS AND FLEXOR HALLUCIS LONGUS

Proximal attachment: *Flexor digitorum longus:* middle one-third of the posterior surface of the tibia. *Flexor hallucis longus:* lateral aspect of the posterior surface of the fibula.

Distal attachment: *Flexor digitorum longus:* passing behind the medial malleolus to attach to the distal phalanges of the four lateral toes. *Flexor hallucis longus:* passing behind the medial malleolus, deep to flexor digitorum longus, to attach to the distal phalanx of the great toe.

Action: *Flexor digitorum longus:* flexion of the four lateral toes; acts weakly in plantar flexion; assists inversion and supination (adduction) of the foot. *Flexor hallucis longus:* flexion of the great toe. Both muscles serve to maintain balance when the body weight is on the forefoot and help stabilize the ankle during walking. Both are vigorously active during the take-off and landing in a vertical two-legged jump.

Palpation: These muscles lie deep to gastrocnemius and soleus and medial to tibialis posterior. Along with tibialis posterior, they comprise the deep posterior compartment of the leg. Flexor digitorum longus may be palpated with the patient lying on the involved side with the knee flexed to 90 degrees and the foot relaxed. Pressure is applied to the posterior aspect of the shaft of the tibia, approximately 3 inches below the joint line. The gastrocnemius is moved laterally to identify the posterior tibia. Pressure is directed laterally to palpate the flexor digitorum longus.

Flexor hallucis longus can only be palpated through the overlying aponeurosis of the gastrocnemius and soleus muscles. The patient lies in the prone position with his foot off the table. Pressure is applied to the posterior fibula at the junction of the middle and lower thirds of the calf, just lateral to its midline.

Pain pattern: *Flexor digitorum longus:* Pain radiates to the middle of the sole of the foot and possibly over the plantar surface of the four lateral toes. Occassionally pain may be experienced at the medial ankle and calf. *Flexor hallucis longus:* Pain radiates to the plantar surface of the great toe and the head of the first metatarsal. Symptoms include pain in the sole of the foot and the plantar surface of the toes, particularly when weight bearing. Hammertoes and/or claw toes may develop as a result of the presence of taut bands in these muscles.

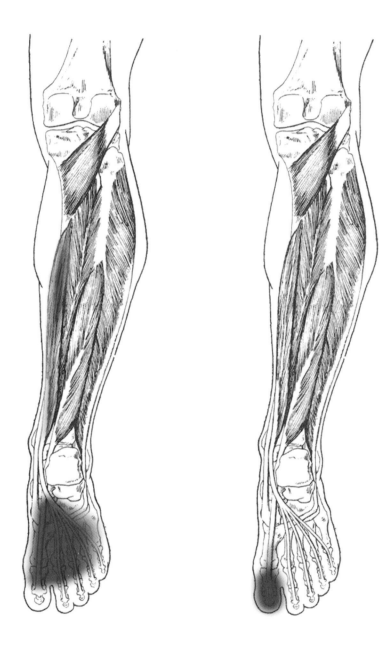

Flexor digitorum longus   *Flexor hallucis longus*

Long flexors of the toes pain pattern

Causative or perpetuating factors: Running on uneven ground, particularly in footwear that does not provide adequate support in the sole or the heel; walking or running on soft sand or on crowned surfaces; wearing shoes that are insufficiently flexible.

Satellite trigger points: Tibialis posterior, extensor digitorum longus, extensor digitorum brevis.

Affected organ system: Genitourinary system.

Associated zones, meridians, and points: Dorsal zone; Foot Tai Yang Bladder meridian; BL 56–59.

Stretch exercise: Sitting with the legs extended in front of you, reach forward, placing the palms of the hands on the plantar surface of the toes. Slowly pull the toes and feet into dorsiflexion. Hold this position for a count of fifteen to twenty.

Strengthening exercise:
1. Using only the toes, grasp a small object such as a marble or pencil.
2. Place a towel on the floor and, using only the toes, try to grasp the towel. Repeat several times.

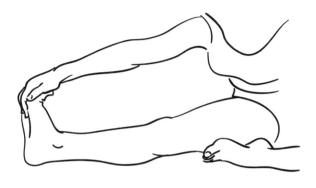

Stretch exercise: Long flexors of the toes

MERIDIAN PATHWAYS

According to the Oriental conception, the body is imbued with an intricate, weblike system of pathways that connect upper and lower aspects of the body as well as connecting superficial regions with internal organ systems. These pathways, or meridians, are connected to one another as well as to a specific organ or system. The often far-reaching effects of acupuncture or acupressure are attributed to the interconnectedness of this system of pathways.

The following basic information on meridian pathways and pairings is included for those who are unfamiliar with rudimentary Oriental anatomy. The interested reader can refer to the following texts to broaden his knowledge in this area:

The Foundations of Chinese Medicine by Giovanni Maciocia (London: Churchill Livingstone, 1989)

Chinese Acupuncture and Moxibustion edited by Cheng Xinnong (Beijing: Foreign Language Press, 1987)

The Manual of Acupuncture by Peter Deadman and Maxin Al-Khafaji with Kevin Baker (East Sussex, England: Journal of Chinese Medicine Publications, 1998)

Meridian name: Hand Tai Yin Lung

Hand/foot pairing: Foot Tai Yin Spleen

Yin/Yang pairing: Hand Yang Ming Colon

Organs through which the meridian passes in its internal pathway: Lung, colon

Muscles traversed by the meridian: Pectoralis major, pectoralis minor, anterior deltoid, biceps brachii, brachialis, brachioradialis, pronator teres, muscles of the thenar eminence

Meridian name: Hand Yang Ming Colon

Hand/foot pairing: Foot Yang Ming Stomach

Yin/Yang pairing: Hand Tai Yin Lung

Organs through which the meridian passes in its internal pathway: Colon, lung

Muscles traversed by the meridian: Extensor pollicis longus, extensor pollicis brevis, extensor carpi radialis longus, extensor digitorum, supinator longus, brachioradialis, triceps brachii, deltoid, supraspinatus, trapezius, sternocleidomastoid, scalenes, orbicularis oris

Meridian name: Foot Yang Ming Stomach

Hand/Foot pairing: Hand Yang Ming Colon

Yin/Yang pairing: Foot Tai Yin Spleen

Organs through which the meridian passes in its internal pathway: Stomach, spleen, large intestine

Muscles traversed by the meridian: Orbicularis oculi, zygomaticus major, orbicularis oris, masseter, temporalis, sternocleidomastoid, pectoralis major, rectus abdominis, external oblique, internal oblique, transversus abdominis, rectus femoris, vastus lateralis, tibialis anterior, extensor digitorum longus

Meridian name: Foot Tai Yin Spleen

Hand/foot pairing: Hand Tai Yin Lung

Yin/Yang pairing: Foot Yang Ming Stomach

Organs through which the meridian passes in its internal pathway: Spleen, stomach, heart

Muscles traversed by the meridian: Extensor hallucis, flexor hallucis brevis, adductor hallucis, tibialis anterior, soleus, gastrocnemius, rectus femoris, sartorius, vastus medialis, adductor longus, adductor brevis, pectineus, iliopsoas, external oblique, internal oblique, transversus abdominis, pectoralis major, pectoralis minor, serratus anterior

Meridian name: Hand Shao Yin Heart

Hand/foot pairing: Foot Shao Yin Kidney

Yin/Yang pairing: Hand Tai Yang Small Intestine

Organs through which the meridian passes in its internal pathway: Heart, small intestine, lung

Muscles traversed by the meridian: Biceps brachii, triceps brachii, pronator teres, palmaris longus, forearm flexors, flexor carpi ulnaris

Meridian name: Hand Tai Yang Small Intestine

Hand/foot pairing: Foot Tai Yang Bladder

Yin/Yang pairing: Hand Shao Yin Heart

Organs through which the meridian passes in its internal pathway: Small intestine, stomach, heart

Muscles traversed by the meridian: Extensor digiti minimi, extensor digitorum, triceps brachii, latissimus dorsi, teres major, infraspinatus, teres minor, posterior deltoid, trapezius, supraspinatus, levator scapulae, scalenes, sternocleidomastoid, masseter, zygomaticus major, temporalis

Meridian name: Foot Tai Yang Bladder

Hand/foot pairing: Hand Tai Yang Small Intestine

Yin/Yang pairing: Foot Shao Yin Kidney

Organs through which the meridian passes in its internal pathway: Bladder, kidney

Muscles traversed by the meridian: Orbicularis oculi, frontalis, occipitalis, splenius capitis, splenius cervicis, semispinalis capitis, semispinalis cervicis, trapezius, levator scapulae, rhomboids, latissimus dorsi, quadratus lumborum, erector spinae group, gluteus maximus, gluteus medius, gluteus minimus, piriformis, semimembranosus, semitendinosus, biceps femoris, soleus, gastrocnemius, tibialis posterior, peroneus brevis, peroneus longus

Meridian name: Foot Shao Yin Kidney

Hand/foot pairing: Hand Shao Yin Heart

Yin/Yang pairing: Foot Tai Yang Bladder

Organs through which the meridian passes in its internal pathway: Bladder, kidney, liver, lung, heart

Muscles traversed by the meridian: Adductor hallucis, flexor digitorum brevis, flexor digitorum longus, tibialis posterior, soleus, gastrocnemius, gracilis, semitendinosus, semimembranosus, sartorius, adductor magnus, iliopsoas, quadratus lumborum, lower abdominals, rectus abdominis, pectoralis major

Meridian name: Hand Jue Yin Pericardium (Heart Constrictor)

Hand/foot pairing: Foot Jue Yin Liver

Yin/Yang pairing: Hand Shao Yang Triple Warmer

Organs through which the meridian passes in its internal pathway: Upper, middle, and lower burners

Muscles traversed by the meridian: Pectoralis major, brachialis, biceps brachii, flexor carpi radialis, palmaris longus

Meridian name: Hand Shao Yang Triple Warmer

Hand/foot pairing: Foot Shao Yang Gall Bladder

Yin/Yang pairing: Hand Jue Yin Pericardium (Heart Constrictor)

Organs through which the meridian passes in its internal pathway: Upper, middle, and lower warmers; bladder

Muscles traversed by the meridian: Extensor digitorum, triceps brachii, deltoid, infraspinatus, supraspinatus, trapezius, sternocleidomastoid, temporalis, orbicularis oculi

Meridian name: Foot Shao Yang Gall Bladder

Hand/foot pairing: Hand Shao Yang Triple Warmer

Yin/Yang pairing: Foot Jue Yin Liver

Organs through which the meridian passes in its internal pathway: Gallbladder, liver

Muscles traversed by the meridian: Orbicularis oculi, temporalis, epicranius, occipitalis, sternocleidomastoid, levator scapulae, trapezius, deltoid, pectoralis major, serratus anterior, external oblique, internal oblique, transversus abdominis, quadratus lumborum, iliopsoas, gluteus minimis, gluteus medius, gluteus maximus, tensor fasciae latae, iliotibial band, vastus lateralis, tibialis anterior, soleus, peroneus brevis, peroneus longus, tibialis posterior, extensor digitorum

Meridian name: Foot Jue Yin Liver

Hand/foot pairing: Hand Jue Yin Pericardium

Yin/Yang pairing: Foot Shao Yang Gall Bladder

Organs through which the meridian passes in its internal pathway: Gallbladder, liver, lungs

Muscles traversed by the meridian: Extensor hallucis longus, extensor hallucis brevis, tibialis anterior, soleus, gastrocnemius, sartorius, gracilis, vastus medialis, adductor magnus, adductor longus, adductor brevis, pectineus, iliopsoas, external oblique, internal oblique, transversus abdominis

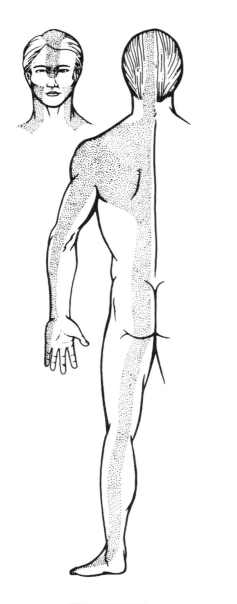

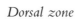

Dorsal zone

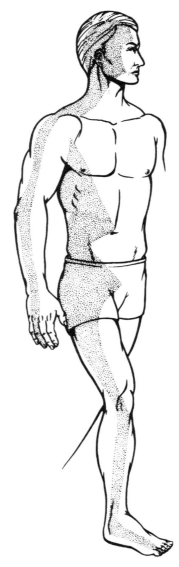

Lateral zone

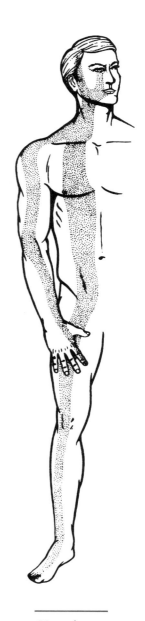

Ventral zone

APPENDIX 2

ON CUTANEOUS ZONES

The concept of zones as developed by Mark Seem, Ph.D., is an intelligent view of the meridian system useful in the treatment of myofascial pain syndromes. The concept of cutaneous zones is part of Dr. Seem's treatment protocol, which is fully described in his book *A New American Acupuncture* (Blue Poppy Press, 1993).

Zones as defined by Dr. Seem are composite representations of associated meridian pathways; a given zone is comprised of the regular meridians, divergent luo, tendinomuscular meridians, and any extraordinary vessels passing through the region. Using the framework of the cutaneous zones one can therefore treat, directly or indirectly, the complex meridian systems contained within a given region.

Dr. Seem has defined three zones through which he treats. The combined hand and foot aspects of Tai Yang (that is, Small Intestine and Bladder meridians, respectively) is named the *dorsal zone* due to their posterior placement in the body. The combined hand and foot aspects of Yang Ming (Colon and Stomach meridians, respectively) is named the *ventral*

zone due to their frontal positioning in the body. The combined hand and foot aspects of Shao Yang, Triple Warmer, and Gall Bladder, respectively, is named the *lateral zone* in accordance with their positioning in the body.

Since constrictions both within the musculature and along meridian pathways both reflect and affect movement within the given region—both on a gross level, as in the ability of the myofascia to produce complete, pain-free movement, as well as on the level of movement of blood and lymphatic fluid, nervous innervation, and so forth—it is essential to release constrictions on every level to ensure healing on all levels. Cutaneous zones, as described by Dr. Seem, provide a guide to the exploration and treatment of related areas as defined from the Oriental perspective.

It is also interesting to note that muscles that are part of a particular zone often develop satellite trigger points in response to the presence of active trigger points in other muscles in that zone. Zones also most commonly contain the referred pain pattern for a muscle lying within a given zone.

COMMONLY USED ACUPOINTS

There are many useful texts delineating the use of acupuncture points (also known as *acupoints*). The interested reader is encouraged to investigate these points and study their applications. The following texts are recommended as sources of acupoint information:

The Foundations of Chinese Medicine by Giovanni Maciocia (London: Churchill Livingstone, 1989)

Chinese Acupuncture and Moxibustion edited by Cheng Xinnong (Beijing: Foreign Language Press, 1987)

The Manual of Acupuncture by Peter Deadman and Maxin Al-Khafaji with Kevin Baker (East Sussex, England: Journal of Chinese Medicine Publications, 1998)

The points listed here are those we have found to be particularly effective in the treatment of patients in whom myofascial constriction is a reflection of organ or system dysfunction. Once a point is selected it should be treated through needling or direct pressure, in conjunction with the treatment of the myofascia.

Additionally, the treatment of local points—acupuncture points located within the affected region—used in conjunction with trigger point release methods can be quite useful to the overall healing of a patient suffering with pain due to myofascial dysfunction.

SOURCE POINTS/ ORGAN POINTS

The acupoints listed here directly treat the given organ. Sensitivity in these points is often a reflection of dysfunction within the organ.

LU 9 for the lungs
CO 4 for the colon
ST 42 for the stomach
SP 3 for the spleen
HE 7 for the heart
SI 4 for the small intestine
BL 64 for the bladder
KI 3 for the kidneys
PC 7 for cardiovascular function
TW 4 for digestive function
GB 40 for the gallbladder
LIV 3 for the liver

HE/SEA POINTS

These acupoints support the relationship between the given organ and the superficial meridian.

LU 5 for the lungs
CO 11 for the colon
ST 36 for the stomach
SP 9 for the spleen
HE 3 for the heart
SI 8 for the small intestine
BL 40 for the bladder
KI 10 for the kidneys
PC 3 for cardiovascular function
TW 10 for digestive function
GB 34 for the gallbladder
LIV 8 for the liver

SUPPORT POINTS

We have found that certain local points, or acupoints located within the region of an organ or system, are useful to the healing of that organ.

LU 1 and 2 support respiration
ST 25 supports the abdomen and treats associated conditions such as those related to digestion and elimination
KI 16 supports the abdomen, kidneys, and pelvis and treats conditions and dysfunctions associated with these organs and regions
KI 21 through 27 support respiration
GB 26 and 27 support and open the pelvis and might be used to treat gynecological and eliminative dysfunctions

BL 23 supports the lower back and kidneys and treats associated conditions
CV 13 and 17 support the upper warmer
CV 12 supports the middle warmer
CV 6 and 10 support the lower warmer
CV 3 and 4 support the lower abdomen, including urinary function, and are used to treat gynecological dysfunction

Distal points, or acupoints located away from the region of an organ or system, are related to that region through the meridian and can be useful in the treatment of that organ or system.

LU 7 supports the head and neck
CO 4 calms and supports the system in general
ST 36 promotes general health and is used to treat abdominal constrictions
SP 6 supports the abdomen and pelvis and treats conditions associated with that region
SP 10 supports gynecological function
SP 21 is the universal luo, or balancing point, of all meridians and is used to support overall health
BL 57 supports and treats the lower back and urinary function
BL 62 supports circulation throughout the back
GB 41 supports the pelvis and treats conditions associated with constrictions within the pelvis

PAIN PATTERN INDEX

This index provides a visual representation of the essential pain patterns in a given region of the body. By referencing this index the reader can quickly determine the various muscles that might be involved in a patient's complaint. The practitioner can then readily review necessary treatment information by turning to the appropriate pages within the body of this text.

It must be remembered that oftentimes several muscles are involved in producing pain in a given region of the body. It is through palpation that the practitioner determines the precise muscle or muscles involved. (The order of muscle placement within this index *does not* indicate frequency of involvement.) It is recommended that each potential pain source be palpated for constrictions and taut bands to ensure that all possibilities have been explored.

HEAD, NECK, AND FACIAL PAIN

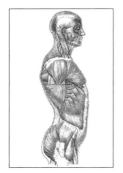

Sternocleidomastoid, p. 32

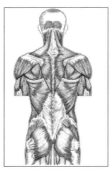

Splenius capitis, p. 40

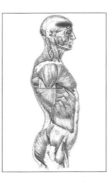

Posterior cervicals (semispinalis capitis), p. 44

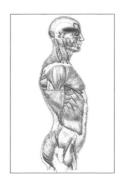

Splenius cervicis, p. 42

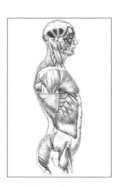

Temporalis, p. 48

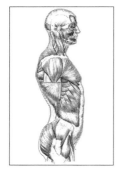

Masseter, p. 50

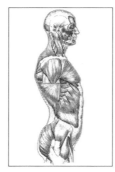

Lateral pterygoid, p. 52

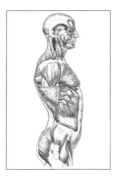

Trapezius, p. 60

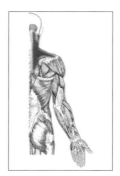

Trapezius, p. 60

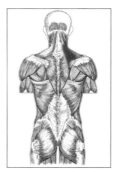

Levator scapulae, p. 62

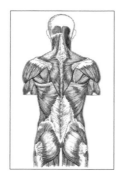

Posterior cervicals (semispinalis cervicis), p. 44

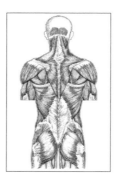

Splenius cervicis, p. 42

POSTERIOR SHOULDER, ARM, AND HAND PAIN

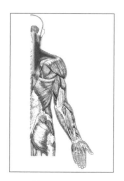

Trapezius, p. 58

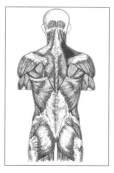

Levator scapulae, p. 62

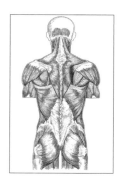

Rhomboids, p. 66

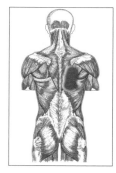

Latissimus dorsi, p. 86

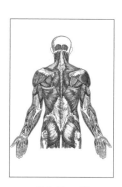

Deltoid, p. 82

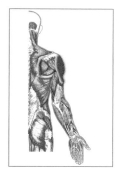

Infraspinatus, p. 98

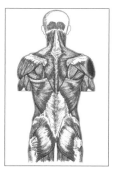

Teres major, p. 90

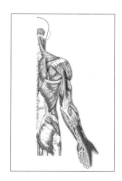

Scalenes, p. 36

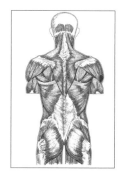

Teres minor, p. 102

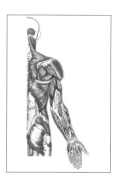

Supraspinatus, p. 94

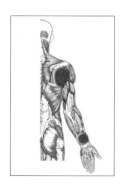

Subscapularis, p. 106

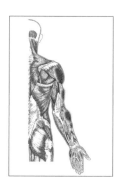

Triceps brachii, p. 114

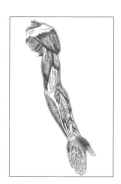

Brachioradialis, p. 118

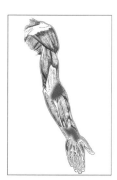

Hand extensors, p. 120

POSTERIOR TORSO AND BUTTOCK PAIN

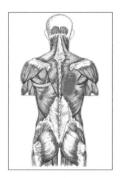

Trapezius, p. 58

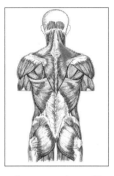

Levator scapulae, p. 62

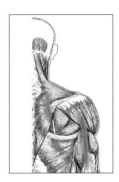

Scalenes, p. 36

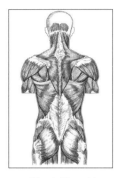

Rhomboids, p. 66

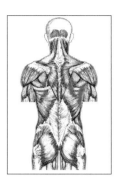

Serratus anterior, p. 68

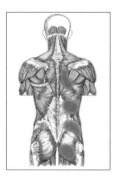

Latissimus dorsi, p. 86

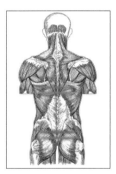

Erector spinae, p. 130

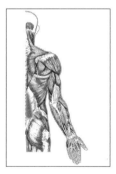

Rectus abdominis, p. 142

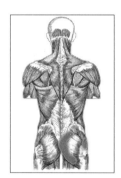

Iliopsoas, p. 138

Gluteus maximus, p. 152

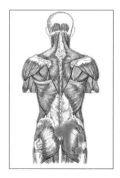

Gluteus medius, p. 156

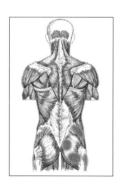

Quadratus lumborum, p. 134

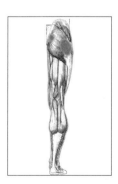

Piriformis, p. 168

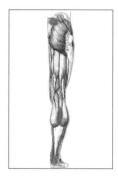

Soleus, p. 198

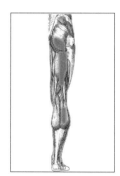

Gluteus minimus, p. 160

POSTERIOR THIGH, LEG, AND FOOT PAIN

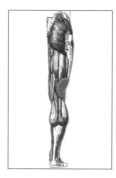

Hamstrings (semitendinosus and semimembranosus), p. 172

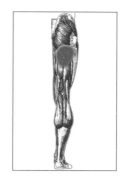

Hamstrings (biceps femoris), p. 172

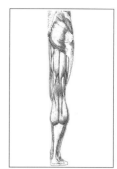

Popliteus, p. 192

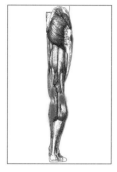

Gastrocnemius, p. 194

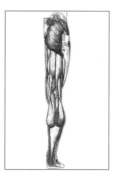

Soleus, p. 198

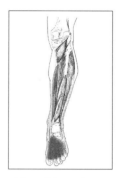

Tibialis posterior, p. 202

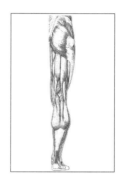

Flexor digitorum longus, p. 216

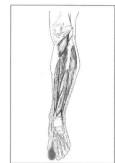

Flexor hallucis longus, p. 216

LATERAL HIP, THIGH, LEG, AND FOOT PAIN

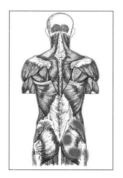

Quadratus lumborum, p. 134

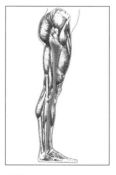

Gluteus minimus, p. 160

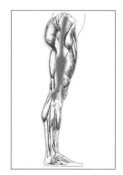

Quadriceps (vastus lateralis), p. 176

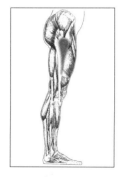

Tensor fasciae latae, p. 164

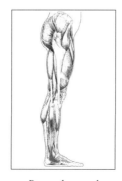

Peroneus longus and peroneus brevis, p. 208

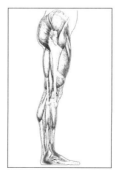

Peroneus tertius, p. 208

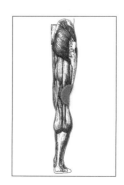

Hamstrings (biceps femoris), p. 172

Anterior Torso, Shoulder, Arm, and Hand Pain

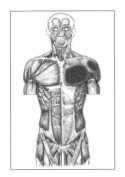

Pectoralis major, p. 78

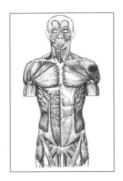

Serratus anterior, p. 68

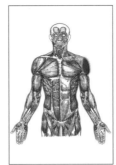

Pectoralis minor, p. 72

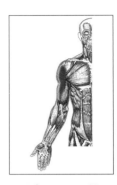

Deltoid, p. 82

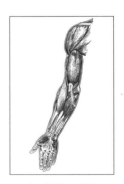

Infraspinatus, p. 98

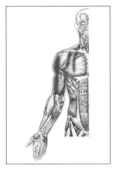

Scalenes, p. 36

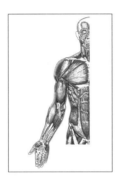

Supraspinatus, p. 94

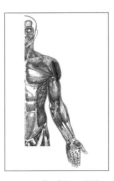

Biceps brachii, p. 110

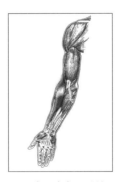

Brachioradialis, p. 118

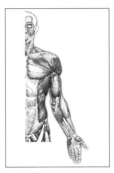

Brachialis, p. 116

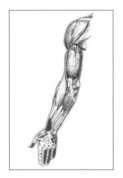

Hand and finger flexors, p. 124

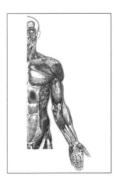

Abdominals (external obliques), p. 146

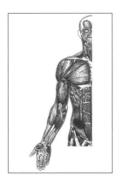

Rectus abdominis, p. 142

ANTERIOR THIGH, LEG, AND FOOT PAIN

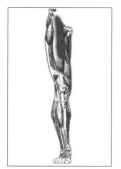

Iliopsoas, p. 138

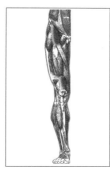

*Adductor longus
and brevis, p. 180*

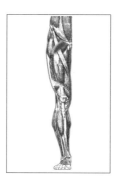

Pectineus, p. 184

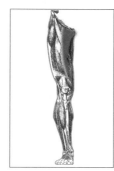

Adductor magnus, p. 180

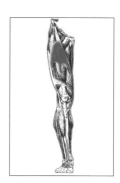

*Quadriceps (vastus
intermedius), p. 176*

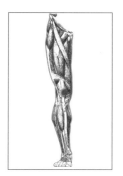

*Quadriceps
(rectus femoris), p. 176*

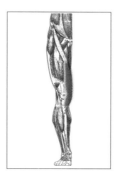

*Quadriceps
(vastus medialis), p. 176*

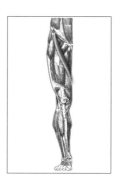

Sartorius, p. 190

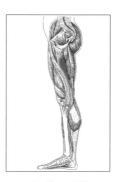

Gracilis, p. 188

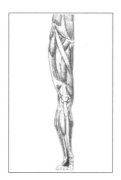

*Extensor digitorum longus,
p. 212*

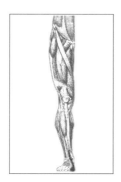

*Extensor hallucis longus,
p. 212*

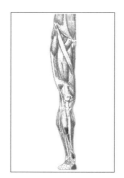

Tibialis anterior, p. 204

Symptom Index

Trigger points in many muscles produce not only pain, but other symptomatology as well. This symptom index is thus provided for easy reference, and is categorized with respect to specific regions of the body. Referencing this index will provide easy access to the muscles that might be the source of various symptomatology. The practitioner can then readily access necessary treatment information by turning to the appropriate pages within the technical body of this text.

Signs and Symptoms Related to the Head, Neck, and Face

Blurred vision: splenius cervicis, 42

Cough (dry): sternocleidomastoid, 32

Dizziness: sternocleidomastoid, 32

Dysmetria: sternocleidomastoid, 32

Eye redness: sternocleidomastoid, 32

Eye tearing: sternocleidomastoid, 32

Headache: splenius cervicis, 42
    sternocleidomastoid, 32
    temporalis, 48
    trapezius, 58

Hearing loss: sternocleidomastoid, 32

Imbalance: sternocleidomastoid, 32

Pain
    ear: masseter, 50
        sternocleidomastoid, 32

    eye: splenius cervicis, 42
        sternocleidomastoid, 32
    facial: masseter, 50
        sternocleidomastoid, 32
        temporalis, 48
    forehead: semispinalis capitis, 44
        semispinalis cervicis, 44
        sternocleidomastoid, 32
    jaw: masseter, 50
        pterygoids, 52
        temporalis, 48
    mouth: pterygoids, 52
    neck: infraspinatus, 98
        levator scapulae, 62
        semispinalis cervicis, 44
        splenius capitis, 40
        splenius cervicis, 42
        trapezius, 58
    occiput: infraspinatus, 98
        semispinalis capitis, 44
        semispinalis cervicis, 44
    temple: semispinalis capitis, 44
        semispinalis cervicis, 44
        sternocleidomastoid, 32
        trapezius, 58
    tooth: masseter, 50
        temporalis, 48
    vertex: splenius capitis, 40
        sternocleidomastoid, 32

Reduced range of motion
    jaw: masseter, 50
        pterygoids, 52

neck: levator scapulae, 62

    semispinalis capitis, 44

    semispinalis cervicis, 44

    splenius cervicis, 42

Sore throat: sternocleidomastoid, 32

    pterygoids, 52

Swallowing difficulties: pterygoids, 52

Tenderness

    posterior head: semispinalis capitis, 44

      semispinalis cervicis, 44

    scalp: sternocleidomastoid, 32

Tinnitus: sternocleidomastoid, 32

    masseter, 50

TMJ dysfunction: masseter, 50

    pterygoids, 52

    temporalis, 48

Tooth sensitivity: masseter, 50

    temporalis, 48

Visual disturbances or blurring:

    splenius cervicis, 42

Signs and Symptoms Related to the Shoulder, Arm, and Hand

Difficulty with

    abduction: deltoid, 82

      subscapularis, 106

      supraspinatus, 94

    reaching back: infraspinatus, 98

      pectoralis minor, 72

      supraspinatus, 94

    reaching up: latissimus dorsi, 86

      pectoralis minor, 72

      supraspinatus, 94

      teres major, 90

    sleeping on the side: infraspinatus, 98

Grip problems

    unreliable: hand and finger extensors, 120

    weak: brachioradialis, 118

      hand and finger extensors, 120

Pain

    elbow, lateral: brachioradialis, 118

      hand and finger extensors, 120

      supraspinatus, 94

      triceps brachii, 114

    elbow, medial: pectoralis major, 78

      triceps brachii, 114

    fingers: hand and finger extensors, 120

      hand and finger flexors, 124

      fourth and/or fifth digits: latissimus

        dorsi, 86

      pectoralis major, 78

      pectoralis minor, 72

      serratus anterior, 68

      triceps brachii, 114

    index: scalenes, 36

  forearm:

    extensor surface: hand and finger extensors, 120

      supraspinatus, 94

      teres major, 90

      triceps brachii, 114

    flexor surface: infraspinatus, 98

    radial aspect: brachioradialis, 118

      infraspinatus, 98

      scalenes, 36

    ulnar aspect: latissimus dorsi, 86

      pectoralis major, 78

      pectoralis minor, 72

      serratus anterior, 68

  hand: hand and finger extensors, 120

    infraspinatus, 98

    latissimus dorsi, 86

    palmaris longus, 124

    pectoralis major, 78

    pectoralis minor, 72

    scalenes, 36

    serratus anterior, 68

    triceps brachii, 114

  midclavicular: sternocleidomastoid, 32

  midscapular: infraspinatus, 98

    levator scapulae, 62

    rhomboids, 66

    scalenes, 36

    trapezius, 58

  scapular: infraspinatus, 98

    latissimus dorsi, 86

    levator scapulae, 62

    rhomboids, 66

serratus anterior, 68

subscapularis, 106

trapezius, 58

triceps brachii, 114

shoulder:

anterior: biceps brachii, 110

deltoid (anterior), 82

infraspinatus, 98

pectoralis major, 78

pectoralis minor, 72

supraspinatus, 94

posterior: deltoid (posterior), 82

latissimus dorsi, 86

serratus anterior, 68

supraspinatus, 94

teres major, 90

teres minor, 102

thumb: brachialis, 116

brachioradialis, 118

scalenes, 36

upper arm:

anterior: biceps brachii, 110

deltoid (anterior), 82

infraspinatus, 98

pectoralis major, 78

pectoralis minor, 72

scalenes, 36

supraspinatus, 94

triceps brachii, 114

posterior: deltoid (posterior), 82

latissimus dorsi, 86

scalenes, 36

subscapularis, 106

supraspinatus, 94

teres major, 90

teres minor, 102

triceps brachii, 114

wrist: subscapularis, 106

Reduced range of motion

abduction: deltoid, 82

pectoralis major, 78

subscapularis, 106

teres major, 90

triceps brachii, 114

adduction: infraspintus, 98

extension of humerus:

deltoid (anterior), 82

infraspinatus, 98

pectoralis minor, 72

supraspinatus, 94

external rotation: subscapularis, 106

flexion of humerus:

deltoid, 82

pectoralis minor, 72

supraspinatus, 94

teres major, 90

internal rotation: infraspinatus, 98

subscapularis, 106

Tenderness

elbow, lateral: triceps brachii, 114

thumb: brachialis, 116

Tennis elbow: brachioradialis, 118

hand and finger extensors, 120

triceps brachii, 114

Trigger finger: hand and finger flexors, 124

Weakness

abduction of humerus: deltoid, 82

arm: scalenes, 36

hand: scalenes, 36

hand grip: brachioradialis, 118

hand and finger extensors, 120

SIGNS AND SYMPTOMS RELATED TO THE CHEST, TORSO, AND ABDOMEN

Bladder pain or dysfunction (including urinary frequency):

adductor magnus, 180

internal oblique, 146

Breathing difficulty: serratus anterior, 68

Digestive dysfunction or pain, including vomiting, nausea, indigestion, fullness, heartburn:

rectus abdominis, 142

external oblique, 146

Gynecological dysfunction or pain, including menstrual cramping, dysmennorhea:

adductor magnus, 180

rectus abdominis, 142

Pain

    abdomen: iliocostalis lumborum, 130

        iliocostalis thoracis, 130

    bladder: adductor magnus, 180

        internal obliques, 146

    breast: pectoralis major, 78

        pectoralis minor, 72

        serratus anterior, 68

    chest: pectoralis major, 78

        pectoralis minor, 72

        scalenes, 36

        serratus anterior, 68

    groin: adductor brevis, 180

        adductor longus, 180

        external oblique, 146

        iliopsoas, 138

        internal oblique, 146

        pectineus, 184

        transversus abdominis, 146

    lumbar, unilateral: iliopsoas, 138

    midclavicular: sternocleidomastoid, 32

    nipple: pectoralis major, 78

        serratus anterior, 68

    pelvic: adductor magnus, 180

    rectal: adductor magnus, 180

    testicular: external oblique, 146

        internal oblique, 146

        transversus abdominis, 146

    thorax, posterior: iliocostalis lumborum, 130

        iliocostalis thoracis, 130

        latissimus dorsi, 86

        rectus abdominis, 142

    vaginal: adductor brevis, 180

        adductor longus, 180

        adductor magnus, 180

SIGNS AND SYMPTOMS RELATED TO THE THIGH, LEG, AND FOOT

Ankle instability: peroneus longus, 208

    peroneus brevis, 208

    peroneus tertius, 208

Ankle tenderness: peroneus longus, 208

    peroneus brevis, 208

    peroneus tertius, 208

Ankle weakness: peroneus longus, 208

    peroneus brevis, 208

    peroneus tertius, 208

    tibialis anterior, 204

Cramps

    calf: gastrocnemius, 194

    foot: extensor digitorum longus, 212

Knee buckling: vastus medialis, 176

Knee, inability to straighten:

    gastrocnemius, 194

    popliteus, 192

    vastus intermedius, 176

Knee stiffness: adductor brevis, 180

    adductor longus, 180

Pain

    ankle: extensor digitorum longus, 212

        gastrocnemius, 194

        gluteus minimus, 160

        tibialis anterior, 204

    calf: gastrocnemius, 194

        gluteus minimus, 160

        semimembranosus, 172

        semitendinosus, 172

        soleus, 198

    foot: extensor digitorum longus, 212

        flexor digitorum longus, 216

        gastrocnemius, 194

        gluteus minimus, 160

    heel: soleus, 194

    knee:

        anterior: adductor longus, 180

            rectus femoris, 176

            vastus medialis, 176

        lateral: biceps femoris, 172

            gluteus minimus, 160

            vastus lateralis, 176

        medial: adductor brevis, 180

            semimembranosus, 172

            semitendinosus, 172

            vastus medialis, 176

        posterior: biceps femoris, 172

            gastrocnemius, 194

            gluteus minimus, 160

popliteus, 192
semimembranosus, 172
semitendinosus, 172
vastus lateralis, 176
leg:
lateral: gluteus minimus, 160
tensor fasciae latae, 164
medial: adductor brevis, 180
shin: tibialis anterior, 204
sole: flexor digitorum longus, 216
flexor hallucis longus, 216
tibialis posterior, 202
thigh:
anterior: iliopsoas, 138
sartorius, 190
vastus intermedius, 176
lateral: biceps femoris, 172
gluteus minimus, 160
tensor fasciae latae, 164
vastus intermedius, 176
vastus lateralis, 176
medial: adductor brevis, 180
adductor longus, 180
adductor magnus, 180
gracilis, 188
sartorius, 190
semimembranosus, 172
semitendinosus, 172
vastus medialis, 176
posterior: biceps femoris, 172
gluteus maximus, 152
gluteus medius, 156
gluteus minimus, 160
piriformis, 168
semimembranosus, 172
semitendinosus, 172
toes: extensor digitorum longus, 212
extensor hallucis longus, 212
flexor digitorum longus, 216
flexor hallucis longus, 216
tibialis anterior, 204
tibialis posterior, 202
Reduced range of motion
abduction: adductor brevis, 180

adductor longus, 180
external rotation: adductor brevis, 180
adductor longus, 180
Toe deformities
claw toes: flexor digitorum longus, 216
hammertoes: flexor digitorum longus, 216

SIGNS AND SYMPTOMS RELATED TO THE HIPS, PELVIS, AND BUTTOCKS

Difficulty with
ascending stairs: vastus intermedius, 176
descending stairs: rectus femoris, 176
soleus, 198
forward bending: erector spinae, 130
lying supine: gluteus medius, 156
rising from a seated position:
gluteus minimus, 160
longissimus thoracis, 130
quadratus lumborum, 134
semimembranosus, 172
vastus intermedius, 176
sidebending: erector spinae, 130
side-lying: gluteus medius, 156
gluteus minimus, 160
tensor fasciae latae, 164
vastus lateralis, 176
sitting: gluteus maximus, 152
gluteus medius, 156
piriformis, 168
semimembranosus, 172
semitendinosus, 172
tensor fasciae latae, 164
standing: gluteus minimus, 160
iliopsoas, 138
piriformis, 168
quadratus lumborum, 134
straightening the knee: popliteus, 192
vastus intermedius, 176
turning in bed: gluteus minimus, 160
quadratus lumborum, 134
walking: gluteus medius, 156
gluteus minimus, 160
piriformis, 168

quadratus lumborum, 134
semimembranosus, 172
semitendinosus, 172
tensor fasciae latae, 164
vastus lateralis, 176
Leg-length discrepancy:
quadratus lumborum, 134
Pain
buttocks: gluteus maximus, 152
gluteus medius, 156
gluteus minimus, 160
iliocostalis lumborum, 130
iliocostalis thoracis, 130
longissimus thoracis, 130
quadratus lumborum, 134
piriformis, 168
semimembranosus, 172
semitendinosus, 172
coccyx: gluteus maximus, 152
groin: adductor brevis, 180
adductor longus, 180
iliopsoas, 138
hip: gluteus maximus, 152
gluteus medius, 156
gluteus minimus, 160

piriformis, 168
quadratus lumborum, 134
tensor fasciae latae, 164
vastus lateralis, 176
iliac crest: gluteus medius, 156
longissimus thoracis, 130
quadratus lumborum, 134
vastus lateralis, 176
lumbar region: gluteus medius, 156
iliopsoas, 138
piriformis, 168
rectus abdominis, 142
posterior thorax: iliocostalis lumborum, 130
iliocostalis thoracis, 130
iliopsoas, 138
rectus abdominis, 142
sacroiliac joint: gluteus maximus, 152
gluteus medius, 156
piriformis, 168
quadratus lumborum, 134
soleus, 198
sacrum: gluteus maximus, 152
gluteus medius, 156
piriformis, 168

BIBLIOGRAPHY

Abbott, Edwin A. *Flatland, A Romance of Many Dimensions.* New York: Harper and Row, 1983.

Baldry, P. E. *Acupuncture, Trigger Points and Musculoskeletal Pain.* Edinburgh/London: Churchill Livingstone, 1989.

Bragdon, Claude. *A Primer of Higher Space.* London: Kessinger, 1999. Originally published 1939.

Calais-Germaine, Blandine. *Anatomy of Movement.* Seattle: Eastland Press, 1993.

Chaitow, Leon. *The Acupuncture Treatment of Pain.* New York: Thorsons, 1983.

Chaitow, Leon. *Palpatory Literacy.* London: Thorsons, 1991.

Denmei, Shudo. *Introduction to Meridian Therapy.* Seattle: Eastland Press, 1990.

DiGiovanna, Eileen and Schiowitz, Stanley, eds. *An Osteopathic Approach to Diagnosis and Treatment.* Philadelphia: Lippincott, 1991.

Dvorak, Jiri and Dvorak, Vaclav. *Manual Medicine* (2nd edition). Stuttgart: Georg Thieme Verlag, 1990.

———. *Manual Medicine Checklist,* Stuttgart: Georg Thieme Verlag, 1990.

Field, Derek. *Anatomy, Palpation, and Surface Markings.* Oxford: Butterworth-Heinemann, 1994.

Goldfinger, Eliot. *Human Anatomy for Artists.* New York: Oxford University Press, 1991.

Gunn, C. Chan. *Treating Myofascial Pain: Intramuscular Stimulation for Myofascial Pain Syndromes of Neuropathic Origin.* Seattle: Multidisciplinary Pain Center, University of Washington Medical School, 1989.

Hammer, Warren. *Functional Soft Tissue Examination and Treatment by Manual Methods (The Extremities).* Gaithersburg, Md.: Aspen, 1991.

Headley, B. J., "EMG and Myofascial Pain," in *Clinical Management,* vol. 10, no. 4. July-Aug., 1990.

Hoppenfeld, Stanley. *Physical Examination of the Spine and the Extremities,* Norwalk, Ct.: Appleton-Century-Crofts, 1976.

Jenkins, David B. *Hollinshead's Functional Anatomy of the Limbs and Back* (6th edition). Philadelphia: Saunders, 1991.

JwingMing, Dr. Yang. *Tai Chi Theory and Martial Power.* Jamaica Plain, Ma.: YMAA Publication Center, 1987.

Kapit, Wynn, and Lawrence Elson. *The Anatomy Coloring Book.* New York: Harper and Row, 1977.

Kendall, Florence, Elizabeth McCreary, and Patricia Provance. *Muscles: Testing and Function.* Baltimore: Williams and Wilkins, 1993.

Lao Tsu. *Tao te Ching.* Translated by Gia-Fu Feng and Jane English. New York: Vintage, 1972.

Maciocia, Giovanni. *The Foundations of Chinese Medicine.* Edinburgh/London: Churchill Livingstone, 1989.

Magee, David J. *Orthopedic Physical Assessment.* Philadelphia: Saunders, 1992.

Mennell, John McMillan. *The Musculoskeletal System.* Gaithersburg, Md.: Aspen, 1992.

Moore, Keith L. *Clinically Oriented Anatomy* (2nd edition). Baltimore: Williams and Wilkins, 1985.

Nielsen, Arya. *Gua Sha: A Traditional Technique for Modern Practice.* New York: Churchill Livingstone, 1995.

Pirog, John E. *The Practical Application of Meridian Style Acupuncture.* Berkeley: Pacific View, 1996.

Platzer, Werner, M.D. *Color Atlas: Textbook of Human Anatomy,* vol I (Locomotor System) (4th edition). New York: Thieme Medical, 1992.

Richer, Paul. *Artistic Anatomy.* New York: Watson-Guptil, 1971.

Schneider, Werner, Hans Spring, and Thomas Tritschler. *Mobility: Theory and Practice.* New York: Thieme Medical, 1992.

Seem, Mark. *A New American Acupuncture.* Boulder: Blue Poppy Press, 1993.

Sieg, Kay, and Sandra Adams. *Illustrated Essentials of Musculoskeletal Anatomy.* Gainsville, Fl.: Megabooks, 1985.

Tortora, Gerard, and Nicholas Anagnostakos. *Principles of Anatomy and Physiology.* New York: Harper and Row, 1981.

Travell, Janet, and David Simons. *Myofascial Pain and Dysfunction: The Trigger Point Manual,* vol I. Baltimore: Williams and Wilkins, 1983.

———. *Myofascial Pain and Dysfunction: The Trigger Point Manual,* vol II. Baltimore: Williams and Wilkins, 1992.

Upledger, John, and Jon Vredevoogd. *Craniosacral Therapy.* Seattle: Eastland Press, 1983.

Wadsworth, Carolyn T. *Manual Examination and Treatment of the Spine and Extremities.* Baltimore: Williams and Wilkins, 1988.

Essentials of Chinese Acupuncture. Compiled by Beijing College of Traditional Chinese Medicine, Shanghai College of Traditional Chinese Medicine, Nanjing College of Traditional Chinese Medicine, and the Acupuncture Institute of Traditional Chinese Medicine. Beijing: Foreign Languages Press, 1980.

Academy of Traditional Chinese Medicine. *An Outline of Chinese Acupuncture.* Beijing: Foreign Languages Press, 1975.